Whispering Currents

Bio-Electric Pathways
for Regeneration and Repair
with the Acuscope & Myopulse

*HOW MULTIPLE DISCOVERIES IN
BIOFEEDBACK, PHYSIOLOGY AND
COMPUTER SCIENCE HAVE MERGED
TO ENHANCE BREAKTHROUGHS IN
ELECTRO-CELLULAR STABILIZATION,
PAIN RELIEF & ACCELERATED
HEALING*

Printed in the U.S.A.
First Edition – August 2016

ISBN-13: 978-1537185385

ISBN-10: 1537185381

CONTENTS

ACKNOWLEDGEMENTS

My initial thanks go to all the pioneers in the field of bio-electricity. Their courage and research have laid the groundwork for the ongoing evolution of healing technologies, helping millions of people on their journey toward wholeness and health.

Secondly, I am grateful to the many teachers I have learned from, both during my college years and those thereafter. Many have been extremely generous with their time and wisdom.

Finally, I want to give out a special thanks to my parents; Abe and Sheila Primack. They were incredibly supportive, patient and made great sacrifices during my search for a career direction while I traveled and experimented, exploring new frontiers in healing. Their insights and guidance played a significant role in my ability and freedom to discover the world as a truth seeker and risk taker.

CHAPTER 1:

FOLLOWING MY INSTINCTS

As a young college bound youth, I never would have imagined that at some point along an interdimensional quantum time-line, I would be exploring the circuit pathways of a breakthrough medical instrument while in the dream state. It wasn't just your run-of-the-mill dream either. I have been to this dimension in other dream and Soul travel ventures where I witnessed numerous medical instruments that have yet to be invented. It was the causal world, a place where past, present and future; appear to somehow stretch together in one continuum beyond linear time and space as we know it. Even though this is exactly what happened, setting all metaphysical rumblings aside, the information to follow is a more intellectual scientific elaboration on my journey in regards to one particular technology. It is my hope that there is value here for those with a passion for healing and service to others.

As a 20 year old in 1980, I, like many young adults, was on a mission to discovering my calling and purpose in life. I was fortunate for growing up in a pleasant rural area of the Catskills where my father was a school teacher. It was while taking his electronics course as a senior in high school that I had my first exposure towards understanding the nature of electricity. At about the same time, it was also somewhat of a jolt when I received a significant electrical shock from an exposed wire connected to a coffee burner, while working in a hotel dining room.

While dabbling in various courses at four different Colleges and Universities between 1977 and 1980, my journey towards figuring out a fitting career path was evolving in unexpected ways as my strengths in science and math encouraged my initial pursuit towards engineering. However, while fully engaged in a liberal arts curriculum at the State University of New York at Albany, I was following an inner nudge about working in the field of psychology. In the summer of 1980, I worked at a telephone crisis center, immersed myself in advanced coursework in Sociology and participated as a volunteer in a galvanic-skin-response Biofeedback study. However, after one disappointing introductory course to social work during the fall semester, I decided to keep searching.

"The Undiscovered Self," an elective college course that I thoroughly loved and appreciated, gave me the space and curiosity to explore my passion for eastern philosophy and other esoteric parapsychology subjects such as the Edgar Cayce and Jane Roberts Material, Jungian Psychology, the teachings of Carlos Castenada and Richard Bach. Coupled with course work in Comparative Religion, Zen Buddhism and Communications theory, I was exposing myself to new frontiers of thinking that fueled my thirst towards self-discovery and other fringe philosophies.

Outside of my required curriculum, I plunged into a book on Homeopathy and found its energetic quantum healing concepts completely and utterly fascinating. I discovered the Paul Twitchell writings of Eckankar and read further about Theosophy, ascended masters, divination, near death and out-of-body experiences. It was then that a strong calling to examine alternative healing as a career awakened for me. I wrote letters of interest to various schools for Natural Medicine in California and New Mexico.

A few months later, following strong visceral gut-level instincts, I blindly settled myself down in Santa Fe, where I began classes at a College for Natural Medicine. Numerous waking-dreams and serendipitous events confirmed to me that I was in the right place at the right time.

While studying at the Santa Fe College of Natural Medicine, I was exposed to Herbology, Nutrition, Applied Kinesiology, Chinese Medicine and Ayurvedic healing traditions. After completing a one-year massage therapy curriculum there, I headed to San Francisco in September of 1982 as a part-time student at the State University of California with the intent of exploring Chinese Medicine as a career path.

I proceeded to interview the administrators at two reputable schools for Traditional Chinese Medicine. They both suggested I should first complete a four-year medical-based training prior to commencing any formal education in Chinese Medicine. I realized that I needed to pursue some kind of Allopathic system of education if I was to accomplish any kind of professional legitimacy in the realm of alternative healing. I visited the library to examine microfiche records of various curriculums and discovered that the course work in Physical Therapy would be the closest undergraduate westernized entry to a holistic medical approach than anything I knew of at that time. I immediately applied and was accepted to the State University of New York at Stony Brook with the intention of completing the requisite course work that would satisfy the requirements to successfully apply and gain acceptance into a Physical Therapy program.

After three semesters of rigorous coursework in chemistry and physics coupled with volunteer work at three different physical therapy clinics; I was accepted into Stony Brook's Physical Therapy program and graduated two years later, in June of 1986 with two Bachelor's degrees; one in Physical Therapy and the other in Liberal Arts. I was fortunate to receive special honors and awards for my original student research project involving the use of Kirlian photography (a fringe energetic evaluation modality invented in Russia) as a method for qualitatively documenting a double blind placebo study of circulation and its' relevance to therapeutic ultrasound.

In the summer of 1986, I started my first job as a physical therapist. My initial rotation was as a Respiratory Therapist in a Cardiac and Intensive care unit at a hospital in the Boston area. I accumulated additional experience working within a traditional rehabilitation capacity in various Boston area home health company's as well starting my own private practice. In the fall of 1989, sensing a strong calling back to Santa Fe, I returned there as a result of experiencing, once again, numerous waking dreams and synchronous serendipitous events that were clearly extraordinary. Within a matter of a few weeks of arriving to Santa Fe, I met a sales rep and trainer for the Acuscope technology, an advanced micro-current electro-therapy device. He had also just relocated to Santa Fe as well. We were surely destined to meet there as if it was orchestrated by some kind of invisible intelligence. He loaned me an original 1979 analogue model of the Electro-Acuscope, which was built into a wooden case that contained an old-fashioned biofeedback meter. As I was about to discover, I had at my disposal, this remarkable energetic medical device that few people or health practitioners knew about or understood.

I proceeded to carry this older model of the Acuscope with me from one home to another, treating patients on my homecare rounds in Santa Fe and the surrounding area. As a result of my prior massage training in Santa Fe coupled with the post graduate manual therapy techniques I learned in Boston, I was able to synergistically integrate my soft tissue training and the probes of this amazing device into a unique approach towards accelerating the healing response in numerous patients'. With regular daily use and practice, this incredible instrument evolved into an intelligent extension of my fingertips, hands and intuition. Soon enough I started to see remarkable results in a wide range of musculo-skeletal and neuromuscular conditions that were unresponsive to other treatment. The responses from my patient case load was so overwhelming that within a couple of months I was compelled to purchase, and at great cost, my own Electro-Acuscope unit, the newer digital model that was used successfully treating injuries at the 1984 Los Angeles Olympics. Shortly thereafter, I also acquired the Electro-Myopulse, its companion technology that worked in symphony with the Acuscope. With the complete updated system in my possession, I opened my own practice while continuing to work part time at the State Penitentiary of New Mexico, where I treated inmates in all levels of security for the remaining two years that I lived in Santa Fe.

I relocated to Boulder Colorado in October of 1991 and settled into my new living arrangements and office quickly and easily. Boulder was a socially and intellectually exciting area with thousands of College students, thousands of young, well educated professionals and hundreds of health practitioners working within the realm of holistic health and alternative healing.

I was able to fit in quite easily and started meeting people of like mind right away. Within a few weeks, I was part of a dynamic private practice located in a historic building on Pearl Street, treating a wide array of patients, many of whom were professional athletes. At this point I was completely and fully engaged in using the Acuscope and Myopulse on virtually every patient I saw. Coupled with manual therapy techniques and Pilates based corrective exercises, the Acuscope and Myopulse system became the mainstay of my success for the next 15 or so years in private practice.

CHAPTER 2

IMAGINING NEW AVENUES FOR HEALING

Throughout history, every conceivable way to help heal the sick has been at the forefront of every culture from ancient shamans to modern neurosurgeons. All methods of healthcare have usually involved doing something 'to the body and mind;' exposing a person to heat, cold, radiation, color, sound, music, fasting, cleansing, surgery and numerous variations of massage techniques, movement and exercise. The list goes on and on; ingesting medicinal herbs, drugs and remedies of all kinds in an effort to elicit a positive healing response from the patient.

Instead of randomly or measurably doing some active or quantitative application to the body, imagine a system that allows the body to engage in a two-way dialogue at the cellular level; a system that both filters out the noise of pathology while whispering corrective electronical signals that enhance self-repair, regeneration and rejuvenation. This breakthrough in accelerated healing has resulted from a synergy of discoveries in cellular physiology coupled with groundbreaking work in programmable array logic solid state circuitry and biofeedback science. I'm sharing this because remarkable and occasionally miraculous results were observed and achieved on a regular basis during the 15 year period when I employed this very technology on patients in my physical therapy practice on a day to day basis. What I observed was not just anecdotal, but measurable. Open wounds would start to close, swelling would quickly subside and range of motion would increase faster and further than any previous treatment. I was fully and completely immersed into my patients' progress and their responses from day to day, observing, modifying and improvising where and when necessary. It was a miraculous journey of healing that I was privileged to be a part of.

For years, while I was in practice treating injured clients, I would meditate and contemplate on what and why I was doing what I did, in an effort to achieve the best possible healing response and outcome with my clients. I was truly eager to have a significant impact on the people I came into contact with. I suppose I wanted to prove to myself that I could be a vehicle for something unique and facilitate a remarkable difference, something more permanent than the bandade of a superficial medication or ice pack.

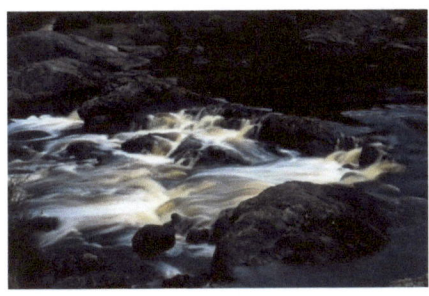 When I attempted to imagine the flow of electrical currents in the body, I often reflected back to when I was a kid, exploring the woods along the river that ran behind the Elementary School where I spent my early years growing up in Mountaindale, New York; a small Hamlet of a few thousand people. Since it was within close walking distance from my home, I would often wander to the river's edge, sheltered by a canopy of oak, maple and birch trees. I was mesmerized by the patterns of water as they carved their way around the many smooth stones, creating a living pattern of color and beauty paired with the symphony of harmonic sounds from a rushing river, the chirping of birds and the gentle breeze in the air. It was a little slice of heaven that I was privileged to experience in my youth. The light and sound were all around and all so noticeable in the natural surroundings, just footsteps from my front door.

When I took up the study of how electrical currents were used in the healing of muscles and connective tissues, I couldn't help but think of how that river would flow around any impediment. It was somewhat of an epiphany when I drew the parallel that an injury, swelling or any inflammatory process for that matter, was as simple as placing a pebble or stone in the flow of the body's natural self-healing signals, like that of a river.

As you read on and learn about biological tissue impedance and other electrical characteristics of all living things, you'll start to realize the importance of un-coupling the impediments to the natural healing currents occurring in the body and why this is of central importance for any self-regulation and self-healing to occur. Ultimately, the human body has the capacity to heal itself if the impediments, both physical and psychological, can be removed, resolved or somehow integrated. How this is accomplished is a coordinated dance of science, skill and intuition.

"If you want to find the secrets of the universe, think in terms of energy, frequency and vibration." - *Nikola Tesla*

"Everything in Life is Vibration"   - *Albert Einstein*

"The human body is made up of electronic vibrations, with each atom and element of the body, each organ and organism, having its electronic unit of vibration necessary for the sustenance of, and equilibrium in that particular organism. Each unit, then, being a cell or a unit of life in it-self, has the capacity of reproducing itself by the first law known as reproduction-division. When a force in any organ or element of the body becomes deficient in its ability to reproduce; that equilibrium necessary for the sustenance of physical existence and its reproduction, that portion becomes deficient in electronic energy. This may come by injury or disease, received by external forces. It may come from internal forces, through lack of eliminations produced in the system or by other agencies to meet its requirements in the body."   - *Edgar Cayce (1928)*

From: "There is a River" by Thomas Sugrue

CHAPTER 3

HISTORICAL CONSIDERATIONS OF HEALING WITH ELECTRICITY

About 100 years ago in the Western world, the study of biochemical interactions became the prevailing paradigm used to explain cellular functions and disease progression. The pharmaceutical industry subsequently became very successful in using this model in developing a series of effective drugs. As medicine became transformed into a huge business during the 20th century, medical treatments became largely based on drug therapies. These pharmaceutical successes have enabled pharmaceutical manufacturers to become wealthy and the dominant influence in medicine. At this point in time the supremacy of the biochemical paradigm and pharmaceutical influences have caused almost all research in medicine to be directed toward understanding the chemistry of the body and the effects that patentable drugs have on altering that chemistry. Yet many biological questions cannot be answered with biochemical explanations alone such as the role of endogenously created electromagnetic fields and electrical currents in the body.

In Western civilization, the first documented use of electricity to manage pain was by the Roman physician Scribonius Largus in 46 AD. He claimed that just about everything from headaches to gout (head to toe) could be controlled by standing on a wet beach near an electric eel. He recorded the use of torpedo fish for treatment of headaches and gout in his Compositiones Medicae.

In 1780, Luigi Galvani, an Italian physician, physicist, biologist and philosopher, discovered animal electricity. He is recognized as the pioneer of bio-electromagnetics. Galvani discovered that the muscles of dead frogs' legs twitched when struck by an electrical spark. This was one of the first forays into the study of bioelectricity.

In 1829, Carlo Matteucci repeated and improved Galvani's experiments on bioelectricity. Matteucci studied mathematics at the University of Bologna and received his doctorate. Matteucci's experiments proved that an electrical current was generated by injured tissue. His work in bioelectricity influenced the research of Emil du Bois-Reymond, who duplicated Matteucci's experiments and discovered the nerve's action potential. In 1843, Reymond observed wound currents in humans where approximately 1 microampere of current, as measured from a wound in human skin.

In 1830, the discovery of alternating current by Faraday opened the door to the development of man-made devices as sources of electricity. Over 10,000 medical practitioners in the United States alone made use of electrotherapeutic modalities until publication of the 1910 Flexner report which stated that there was no scientific basis for Electromedicine at that time. Dr. Flexner's report was originally prepared by the American Medical Association and sponsored by the Carnegie Endowment for the Advancement of Teaching. Perhaps they had other ideas in mind considering Louis Pasteur's germ theory of disease and their investment in the pharmaceutical industry.

In 1882, researchers were able to measure the current generated by the amputated stump of a child's fingertip. These stump currents were found to be within the range of 10-30 microamps per square centimeter. These findings were repeated by several researchers over the years that followed.

In 1924, Hans Berger, using an electroencephalogram, a device he made himself, was the first to record and measure electrical frequencies transmitted by the human brain.

In 1929, Georges Lakhovsky, a Russian engineer, wrote; "The Secret of Life." In it he stated that life is the dynamic equilibrium of all cells, the harmony of multiple radiations which react upon one another, while disease is the oscillatory disequilibrium of cells, originating from external causes. Lakhovsky postulated that every living being emits electro-magnetic radiations and the nucleus of a living cell could be compared to an electrical oscillating circuit. The nucleus consisted of tubular filaments, chromosomes and mitochondria, insulating material and filled with conducting fluid containing all the mineral salts found in sea water. These filaments are comparable to oscillating circuits endowed with capacitance and self-inductance and therefore, capable of oscillating according to a specific frequency. Lakhovsky believed that the fight between the living organism and microbes is fundamentally a war of radiations. If the radiations' of the microbe wins, the cell ceases to oscillate and death is the ultimate result. If, on the other hand, the radiations' of the cell is supported, the microbe is killed and health is preserved. Broadly speaking, health is equivalent to oscillatory equilibrium while disease is characterized by oscillatory disequilibrium.

In his research, Lakhovsky explained that all living cells (plants, people, bacteria, etc.) possess attributes which normally are associated with electronic circuits. These cellular attributes include resistance, capacitance and inductance. Not only do all living cells produce and radiate oscillations of high frequencies but also receive and respond to oscillations imposed upon them from outside sources. The energies of living cells he described make direct energetic communication between life forms possible. Lakhovsky stated: *"electrical energy plays a fundamental part in the organization of the growth and function of protoplasm. Man is a radio-electrical mechanism. When life ends, radiation ends. It is clear that radiation produces the electric current that operates the organism as a whole, producing memory, reason, imagination, emotion, the special senses, secretions, muscular action, the response to infection, and normal growth, all of which are governed by the electrical charges that are generated by the short-wave or ionizing radiation in protoplasm."*

In 1936 Dr. Crile stated in his book, "The Phenomena of Life," that all living cells are electrical and function as a system of generators, inductance lines and insulators. The role played by radiation and electricity in living processes is no more mysterious in man than in batteries.

At the same time in the 1930's; Raymond Royal Rife was conducting his own medical trials with his 'frequency instrument'. He discovered when looking at cancer cells under a microscope, that they changed their size and form. After he exposed them to certain frequencies of radio waves they were destroyed. Rife went on to cure 1,000+ patients of cancer before the medical industry raided his labs and destroyed his machines.

In 1931, Dr. Otto Warburg, MD, PhD, won the Nobel Prize in Medicine/Physiology for his "discovery of the nature and mode of action of the respiratory enzyme." His pioneering work paved the way for the field of biochemistry and he spent most of his life doing cancer research. According to Warburg, cells maintain a voltage across their membrane, which is analogous to the voltage of a battery. He found that healthy cells have a measurable voltage from 70-100 millivolts, with the heart cell having the highest (upwards to 90-100 millivolts). Warburg found that the constant stress of modern life along with the toxicity of the environment coupled with aging contributed to a measurable drop in cellular voltage. People with chronic illnesses and chronic fatigue had diminished cellular voltages from 30-50 millivolts. Cancer patients displayed the lowest cellular voltage at 15-20 millivolts and less. You've probably never heard of someone with heart cancer. Perhaps it has something to do with the heart having the highest cellular voltage of any cell in the body. He summarized that optimal health is part of an energy game that takes place at the cellular level.

From 1935-1957, Harold Saxton Burr was Professor of Anatomy at the Yale University School of Medicine. Burr was a member of the faculty of medicine for over forty-three years. From 1916 to the late 1950's, he and his colleagues published more than ninety-three scientific papers including numerous studies on the Bio-electric nature of living systems, many of which were published in the Yale Journal of Biology & Medicine and the American Journal of Obstetrics & Gynecology. In 1935 he published (with F. S. C. Northrop) "The Electro-Dynamic Theory of Life" and (with C. T. Lane) "Electrical Characteristics of Living Systems". Burr's research contributed to the electrical detection of cancer cells, experimental embryology, neuroanatomy and the regeneration and development of the nervous system. His studies on the bio-electrics of ovulation and menstruation eventually led to the marketing of fertility-indicating devices.

Upon decades of work that Burr carried out, he contended that the electro-dynamic fields of all living things, which can be measured and mapped with standard voltmeters, modify and control each organism's development, health and mood. Burr discovered that every living thing generates an electro-dynamic field that serves as a matrix directing its growth. He called these living fields "L-fields" or "fields of life," which are the basic blueprints of all life on this planet. The L-field maintains the arrangement of whatever material is within it, no matter how often that material changes. Burr believed that, since measurements of L-field voltages can reveal physical and mental conditions, doctors should be able to use them to diagnose illness before symptoms develop, and so would have a better chance of successful treatment.

In his book; "Blueprint for Immortality", Dr. Burr wrote: *"The following theory may then be formulated. The pattern or organization of any biological system is established by a complex electro-dynamic field which is in part determined by its atomic physio-chemical components and which in part determines the behavior and orientation of those components. This field is electrical in the physical sense and by its properties relates the entities of the biological system in a characteristic pattern and is itself, in part, a result of the existence of those entities. It determines and is determined by the components. More than establishing a pattern, it must maintain that pattern in the midst of a physio-chemical flux. Therefore, it must regulate and control living things. It must be the mechanism, the outcome of whose activity is wholeness, organization, and continuity."*

Electro-dynamic fields are invisible, intangible and it is difficult to visualize them. But a crude analogy may help to show what these fields of life do and why they are so important. Most people who have taken high school science will remember that if iron filings are scattered on a card held over a magnet, they will arrange themselves in the pattern of the 'lines of force' of the magnet's field. And if the filings are thrown away and fresh ones scattered on the card, the new filings will assume the same pattern as the old. Something like this happens in the human body. Its molecules and cells are constantly being torn apart and rebuilt with fresh material from the food we eat. But, thanks to the controlling L-fields, the new molecules and cells are rebuilt as before and arrange themselves in the same pattern as the old ones. Until modern instruments revealed the existence of these controlling L-fields, biologists were at a loss to explain how our bodies 'keep in shape' through ceaseless metabolism and changes of material. Now the mystery has been solved: the electro-dynamic field of the body serves as a matrix or pattern which preserves the 'shape' or arrangement of any material poured into it, however often the material may be changed. For nearly half a century, the consequences of this theory have been subjected to rigorously controlled conditions and met with no contradictions."

In 1941, Albert Szent-Gyorgyi (a physiologist who won the Nobel Prize in Medicine in 1937) published an article entitled, "Towards a New Biochemistry," which suggested that energy, in living systems, may be transmitted by conduction bands. Within the structure of the living cell membrane are cellular constituents that are organized and resemble the structure of *liquid crystals*.

Gyorgyi suggested that the electron flow would be similar to photosynthesis, in which a kind of waterfall of electrons cascaded step by step down a staircase of molecules, losing energy with each bounce. The main difference was that in protein semi-conduction, the electrons' energy would be conserved and passed along as information, instead of being absorbed and stored. He conjectured that protein molecules, each having a sort of slot or way-station for mobile electrons, might be joined together in long chains so that electrons could flow in a semi-conducting fashion over long distances without losing energy and that many parts of the cell was regular enough to support this semi-conduction. His ideas were almost completely ignored at the time. When Gyorgyi studied Collagen, the most abundant protein in the human body, he discovered that it behaved like a semiconductor (a material that has electrical conductivity due to flowing electrons). He also discovered that the water surrounding the collagen also conducted protons. Gyorgyi theorized that electron and proton conduction in the molecular and aqueous framework of the body could provide the understanding of rapid energetic communication networks in the body and that these systems may be compromised in cancer and other chronic diseases.

Modern research has confirmed these ideas and we now know that many of the molecules in our bodies do behave like semiconductors, and devices made from semiconductor materials are the foundation of all modern electronics. In his book: "Bioelectronics: A study in cellular regulation, defense, and cancer," Gyorgi postulated that the cell is a machine driven by energy. He stated that the living system may be permeated by an 'invisible fluid,' where the particles of 'electrons' are more mobile than molecules and carry energy, charge and information; acting as the fuel of life. These electrons may help to connect molecules to meaningful structures and may also be responsible for the subtlety of biological reactions. Gyorgyi, also the discoverer of Vitamin C, felt that the problem with cancer is not that cells are replicating themselves, since replication is natural. The abnormality may be within faulty bio-electronic switching mechanisms, which cannot turn off the replicating process. His studies of the electrical effects on implanted tumors in mice at the Mount Sinai School of medicine have suggested that electrical currents may enhance cancer-killing effects of conventional chemotherapy. Mice with melanoma that were exposed to special electrical currents and chemotherapy survived nearly twice as long; than cancer-ridden mice given chemotherapy alone. His mouse melanoma experiments' suggest that electronic currents and electromagnetic fields may be able to manipulate these abnormal electronic switching mechanisms. Other Internal structures, including mitochondria can be viewed as tiny batteries or electrical power sources. Similar to other researchers before him, the implication is that there may be electronic switching and transmission systems within and between cells.

In 1945, Dr. D.D. Eley, Professor and Chair of physical chemistry at the University of Nottingham, investigated the electrical activity of large molecules with possible applications in enzyme action. His research showed that proteins have strongly linked to them a great amount of electron donors and also behave as semiconductors. Eley postulated efficient charge transfer through DNA and that the DNA molecule might behave as a one-dimensional aromatic crystal with electron conductivity.

In the early 1950s, Reinhold Voll, a German physician, developed testing instruments for finding acupuncture points electrically. Although his device was primarily used for electro-diagnostic testing, it was also used to apply therapeutic micro-current to the body. He was successful in finding acupuncture points electrically and demonstrated that these points, known to Chinese acupuncturists for millennia, had a different resistance to a tiny electrical current passing through the body, than did the adjacent tissues. Many other researchers have also verified that electrical conductance at the acupuncture points is significantly greater than the surrounding tissue.

Voll began a lifelong search to identify correlations between disease states and changes in the electrical resistance of various acupuncture points. He thought that if he could identify electrical changes in certain acupuncture points associated with certain diseases, then he might be able to identify those diseases more easily, or earlier, when treatment intervention was likely to be more effective. Voll was successful in identifying many acupuncture points related to specific conditions and published a great deal of information about using acupuncture points diagnostically. (Until Voll, these points had been used mainly for treatment). He found, for example, that patients with lung cancer had abnormal readings on the acupuncture points referred to as lung points. Changes also occurred in the electrical conductance of the acupuncture points supplying musculoskeletal structures that are inflamed. Voll discovered that certain acupuncture points showed abnormal readings when subjects were reacting allergically. He made several serendipitous discoveries related to "allergy" testing. He noted some unusual readings on certain acupuncture points when a patient had a bottle of medicine in his pocket. He could remove the bottle and consistently get different readings when the bottle was in his pocket compared to when it was not. At first he was baffled as to how a closed bottle of medicine outside the body could affect the acupuncture readings. It was even more baffling when he discovered that the glass bottle of medicine could change the readings when it was in contact anywhere along the closed electric circuit involved with the testing procedure. Voll and his colleagues then began to identify the nature of this strange phenomenon. They inserted a metal plate into the circuit and demonstrated that many substances that preclude changes in acupuncture point readings when ingested could produce the same changes when placed on the plate (even in closed glass bottles). They assumed that there must be some kind of electro-magnetic energy being emitted from the substances, and that these energy fields somehow traveled along the electric circuit to the body (perhaps like the energy waves representing a person's voice travels along the electric circuitry of a telephone line).

Dr. William Tiller, past president of the Material Science Department at Stanford University, believed that the skin had a uniform conductance, and he set out to prove that Voll's work was a farce. What he found, however, was that the points on the body that had been mapped out thousands of years ago by the Chinese did, in fact, have a lower resistance than the rest of the skin. He subsequently agreed with Dr. Voll that, where the readings were higher (higher conductance meaning lower resistivity at that point) there was an inflammation of the area associated with that point. This inflammation caused an increase of ions which enhanced the flow of electrons. Conversely, when the reading was low (low conductance meaning higher resistivity) there was a degeneration of the area associated with that point. Degeneration caused a decrease in ion concentrations that

26

hindered the flow of electrons. This pattern of associating low readings with degeneration was studied by Drs. S.G. Sullivan, MD, J.T.Martinoff, MD, PhD, D.W. Eggleston, DDS, and R.J. Korenig, MD who applied it in their research on confirmed lung cancer patients. Their study validated that the lower readings on the lung meridian were indeed reflected in the confirmed cancer patients and not on the healthy patients.

The June 1996 issue of the Institute of Engineers magazine published several articles on acupuncture and the clinical aspects of EAV. Their abstracts confirm that the technology works. A quote from Susan Stockton's book The Terrain is everything states: "Homeostasis is the body's balancing mechanism. When the body is out of balance, energy can no longer flow freely. Energy blockages set up and that leads to disease conditions. Health, in a very real sense, is energy, energy flowing freely through the body without obstruction." We can conclude from Stockton's comment that health is the easy flow of nutrition, air, water, thoughts and energy into and out of the body. A disruption of that flow would then be disease. Being symptom-free is not a sign of health.

In 1972, Kenneth S. Cole, in his book "Membranes Ions and Impulses," discussed the structure of living membranes. He suggested that the bio-molecular leaflet of phospholipids in the cell membrane assumed a structure that resembled that of liquid crystals.

Ross Adey, M.D. (1922-2004) chaired or participated in sessions dealing with the psychophysiologic effects of weak magnetic fields and communications between cells at almost every Congress since their inception. The more than 400 papers, chapters and books he has authored are devoted to interests in electromagnetic field interactions with biological

27

systems, cell membrane organization and intercellular communication, organization of cerebral systems and cellular mechanisms, bioengineering computer applications in medical imaging, physiologic data analysis, and modeling of brain mechanisms and systems. His superb achievements in these areas have been acknowledged by his peers with numerous honors here and abroad, including Fellowship in the American Academy of Arts and Sciences as well as the Institute of Electrical and Electronic Engineers, the D'Arsonval Award from the Biolelectromagnetics Society, the Sechenov medal of the Russian Academy of Medical Sciences and his appointment as distinguished visiting Professor of the Royal Society of Medicine in the U.K. Ross Adey is perhaps best known for the "Adey Window" which has significantly increased our understanding of how the biological effects of feeble electromagnetic fields are mediated.

With contributions to all phases of electroencephalography, from the design of surface and invasive electrodes to signal analysis, Adey was the first to use general purpose digital computers in the analysis of the EEG. His research led to the production of brain maps of electrical activity and the first normative library of such maps. He served on White House Advisory Committees, addressed Congress, delivered keynote addresses (including for the Royal Society of Medicine), and chaired the National Council on Radiation Committee on Extremely Low Frequency Electromagnetic Fields. His many honors include Distinguished Professor, Royal Society of Medicine, and he was a recipient of the Hans Selye Award. He is perhaps best known for discovering, with Suzanne Bawin, the first non-thermal effect of electromagnetic radiation during the 1970s: They showed how ELF-modulated Radio Frequency signals can lead to the release of calcium ions from cells. While at the

Brain Research Institute at the University of California, Los Angeles, Adey worked with the Department of Defense on Project Pandora, the super-secret program that sought a way to use electromagnetic radiation for mind control. In the late 1970s, Adey set up a new lab at the VA Hospital in Loma Linda, CA, where he carried out studies on the role of power frequency EMFs in the promotion of cancer and later, on the potential cancer risks following exposure to cell phone radiation.

In 1993, Adey extensively described in his publications that the application of weak electromagnetic fields of certain windows of frequency and intensity act as first messengers by activating glycoprotein receptors in the cell membrane. Electrical oscillations of the right frequency and amplitude can alter the electrical charge distribution in cell receptors causing the cell receptors to undergo conformational changes just as if the receptor was activated by a chemical signal. The electrical properties of cell receptor-membrane complexes would allow cells to scan incoming frequencies and tune their circuitry to allow them to resonate at those particular frequencies. Adey and other researchers reported that one effect of the application of weak electromagnetic fields is the release of calcium ions inside of the cell. Adey documented that cells respond constructively to a wide range of frequencies including frequencies in the extremely low frequency (ELF) range of 1-10 Hz a range of frequencies known as the Schumann resonance frequencies that are naturally produced in the atmosphere. Adey reported that certain frequency bands between 15-60 Hz have been found to promote cancers, alter cell protein synthesis, mRNA functions, immune responses and intercellular communication.

CHAPTER 4

THE MODERN EVOLUTION OF MICROCURRENT ELECTRO-THERAPY

Transcutaneous electrical nerve stimulation (TENS) came on the scene in the 1970s following Melzack and Wall's introduction of the Gate Control Theory of pain in 1965 in which counter stimulation could effectively close the gate to peripheral pain messages attempting to ascend spinal pathways to the brain. TENS stimulation is typically applied at a level of 60 or more milliamperes of current. Many years later, microcurrent electrical therapy (MET) attempted to alter or eliminate the pain message by inducing normalization of neural function, as well as healing at the pain site, as opposed to serving as a counter-irritation analgesic as that found with TENS.

Following closely behind TENS was the introduction, in the 1980s, of electromagnetic bone healing devices that are utilized to heal non-union fractures. This allowed physicians to promote healing of non-union fractures that previously necessitated amputation.

So, from slow beginnings in the latter half of the 20th century, we now have hundreds of FDA approved electrical devices. Some stimulate muscle contraction so that people with paralyzed muscles can maintain muscle tone in unused limbs thus preventing atrophy. Other disabled people use them in learning to walk again, or in developing new skills in using their arms or hands, for example.

Various electrical stimulators are now widely implanted in the body, such as the cardiac pacemaker, electrical stimulators in various parts of the brain to prevent such things as fine tremor of the hands or whole body seizures, and now for depression. Dorsal column stimulators implanted along the spinal cord interdict pain from various etiologies. We have had electro-acupuncture since the early 1970's when it was introduced from China via Hong Kong. Many contemporary acupuncturists use some form of electro-medical treatment delivered to the acupuncture points because it is safer, faster, more effective, and provides longer lasting results. Many acupuncturists prefer electrical modalities to needles for these reasons and that it avoids the fear of needles some people experience.

Most of the published research on the effects of microcurrents on soft-tissue injury; have described the accelerated healing of skin ulcers and associated suppression of bacterial growth. One of the first studies documenting the positive effects of micro-current stimulation on wound healing and bone fractures was the team of Wolcott, et al, in 1969. These researchers applied stimulation in the range of 200 - 800 micro-amps to a wide variety of wounds. A control group was treated with ordinary wound care methods. The treated group showed 200 - 350% faster healing rates than controls, with stronger tensile strength of scar tissue and antibacterial effects in infected wounds. In 1975, Gault and Gatens used a similar procedure on patients with diagnosis including: quadriplegia, CVA, brain tumor, peripheral vascular disease, burns, diabetes, fracture and amputation. Their results demonstrated healing times in the treated group about half that of the controls. Many other researchers followed variations of these models and published similar results.

Even though microcurrent therapy first gained popularity in the treatment of wounds in the 1980's, it became an accepted procedure with orthopedic surgeons to treat nonunion fractures and other significant soft tissue injuries. In 1984, William Stanish, M.D., physician for the Canadian Olympic team, found that implanted electrodes delivering 10-20 microamps of electrical current hastened recovery from ruptured ligaments and tendons. Using microcurrent, Stanish shortened the normal 18-month recovery period to only 6 months.

Cheng et al (1982) In a study with important implications for microcurrent electrotherapy, examined the effects of electric currents of various intensities on three variables critical to the healing process: At 500 micro-amps, ATP generation (or cellular energy production) increased about 500% and amino acid transport was increased by 30 to 40 percent above control levels using 100 to 500 micro-amps. When currents were increased to the milliampere range, ATP generation was depleted, amino acid uptake was reduced by 20-73 percent and protein synthesis was inhibited by as much as 50%. These findings suggest that the higher milliamp currents inhibit healing whereas the lower microampere currents promote healing. The idea here is that less is often better, similar to the laws of Homeopathy. The conclusion is that attempting to bombard the body with too much energy can end up being counterproductive. Additional studies with isolated tissue or cultured cells provide compelling evidence that the intracellular rates of ATP re-synthesis, protein synthesis and DNA replication are increased as a result of direct electrical stimulation of human fibroblasts.

In 1983, "Biologically Closed Electric Circuits," was written, covering more than 20 years of research by Dr. Bjorn Nordenstrom, head of diagnostic Radiology at Stolkholm's Karolinska Institute. He won the Nobel Prize for his x-ray guided needle biopsies while exploring the use of electric currents to treat cancer. Utilizing electric currents, Nordenstrom was successful in producing complete remission from various types of cancers metastatic to the lung in a significant number of cases considered untreatable by other cancer therapies. Nordenstrom proposed that bioelectricity is conducted through the micro-capillary circulatory system in the body and bioelectrical circuits are part of an undiscovered circulatory system. Nordenstrom claimed to have discovered an unknown universe of electrical activity in the human body, the biological equivalent of electrical circuits. He believed that the body's electrical circuits become switched on by injury, infections', tumors', and even by the normal activity of the body's organs. When injury occurs, a positive charge builds up in the area and sets up a voltage potential difference, which serves as a "bio-electric battery" waiting for the switch to be turned on. This bioelectricity is then switched on by a change in the electrical properties of capillary membranes. As the membranes become less permeable to the flow of ions and more electrically insulated, *the flow of intrinsic bioelectricity is forced to take the path of least resistance*, which is through the bloodstream. These circuits are switched on by the normal activity of the body's organs; voltages build and fluctuate; electric currents course through arteries and veins and across capillary walls, drawing white blood cells and metabolic activity.

Nordenstrom, like other bio-energetic researches, agrees that disturbances in the bioelectrical network of the body may be involved in the development of cancer and other diseases and this electrical system represents the very foundation of the healing process. Every human thought and action is accompanied by the production of electrical signals along the fibers of the nervous system. Indeed, life wouldn't exist at all without a constant flow of ions across the membranes of cells. If Nordenstrom is right, these circuits may explain many fundamental regulatory processes in the human body, and even the seemingly inexplicable therapeutic effects.

Further studies have demonstrated the effects of microcurrent in accelerating healing of bone, tendon repairs, and collagen remodeling. In 1991, The Nobel Prize in Physiology or Medicine was awarded jointly to Erwin Neher and Bert Sakmann for their discoveries concerning the detection of subtle electrical currents and single ion channels in all types of cell membranes throughout the body. This study opened the way for greater understanding of the mechanisms through which externally applied currents can affect organic functions.

With Gyorgyi's idea in mind, Dr Robert Becker, a highly regarded orthopedic surgeon in the 1990's, postulated an analog-coded information system that was closely related to the nerves but not necessarily located in the nerve fibers themselves. Becker theorized that this system used semi-conductive direct currents and that, either alone or in concert with the nerve impulse system, regulated growth, healing, and other basic processes essential in maintaining health.

Becker, twice nominated for the Nobel Prize, pioneered the application of electrotherapy to stimulate the body's innate capacity for tissue repair and regeneration. Becker developed the methods, which are used today for treating non-union fractures with electricity. Becker theorized that a naturally occurring "current of injury" is measurable in the body and hypothesized that this current was conducted by the nerve sheaths (myelin) surrounding neurons (nerves) to an area of injury, thus triggering tissue repair and regeneration.

Becker's work also uncovered new mechanisms of information transmission within the nervous system that may be part of a healing feedback loop. This system seems to involve the Glial and Schwann cell network that surrounds most of the nerves throughout the body. Glial and Schwann cells were originally thought to be strictly nutritive to the nearby nerves. But Becker's work suggests that both types of cells may be information transmitters. Becker's studies also indicate that the information is transmitted along the Glial and Schwann cells, via slow analog changes in direct current rather than via rapid changes in the digital pulse code of action potentials as traditionally observed in nerve transmission.

Becker also looked at cellular mechanisms from the perspective of electronics and cybernetic communication systems. He found that at the level of the single cell, micro-crystalline and other cellular sub-elements may be involved in the modulation of intracellular electrical currents in a way similar to semiconductor circuitry. Certain cellular elements, such as membranes, can be seen to act as capacitors.

Semi-conduction was a laboratory curiosity in the 1930's. In our present time, modern computers, satellites and all the rest of our solid-state electronics would be impossible without semiconductors. Semi-conduction normally occurs only in materials having an orderly molecular structure, such as crystals, in which electrons can move easily from the electron cloud around one atomic nucleus to the cloud around another.

Arthur C. Guyton, M.D. in his classic, "Textbook of Medical Physiology;" discusses the cell membrane as a capacitor. Guyton states that the alignment of electrical charges on the two sides of the cell membrane is exactly the same process that takes place when an electrical capacitor becomes charged with electricity. "In the cell membrane, the lipid matrix of the membrane is the dielectric, much as mica and mylar are frequently used as dielectrics in electrical capacitors."

An understanding of the digital and analog systems of the body can be used to explain the differing effects of; milliamp and microamp therapy. The more primitive system, the analog system, consists of subtle direct currents, which exist in the brain and perineural (conductive) system of the body. The digital system consists of alternating currents produced by activity of nerves and muscle. According to Becker, Salamanders, lizards, and other simple creatures, easily regenerate whole limbs and organs due to the analog system, which controls healing. This system also allows birds and other migratory animals to guide themselves by direct contact with the magnetic fields of the earth. Humans have limited powers of regeneration because our bodies favor a highly developed digital nervous system, which allows greater abilities in complex motor skills and conscious thought.

A salamander can regenerate a third of its total body mass including brain, heart and spinal cord. Becker learned that if the same electrical parameters (which he had measured) were applied to other animals, a significant amount of regeneration could take place. Dr. Becker was able to experimentally cause frogs and rats to regenerate amputated limbs through DC electro-stimulation, a feat they are unable to do in nature. The rat regrew half of its amputated front leg from shoulder to elbow, and a frog regrew its entire front leg right down to the individual digits of its webbed feet. With current in the nano-ampere range (billionths of an ampere), Becker was able to clear up grossly infected wounds; osteomyelitis in just seven days, where antibiotics had failed completely. Becker's most astonishing discovery was that, under the influence of an appropriately applied direct current, in the micro-ampere range, certain cells are capable of dedifferentiation. He found that, in frogs, mature, fully differentiated cells are able to retrogress to an embryonic form, then; re-differentiate into whatever cell types are needed for complete regeneration.

The discrete pulses of milliamp stimulation resemble the digital activity of the nervous system and therefore can interact with it to temporarily suppress pain. **Micro-currents, on the other hand, more closely match the analog systems of the body**. If indeed it is the primitive DC systems of the body that modulate healing, this may offer an explanation for the documented healing acceleration effects of micro-current treatment.

In his 2001 book; "Energy Medicine: The Scientific Basis," James Oschman, PhD, sees the entire body as one interconnected organism, a living matrix of communication analogous to the nervous system. "Each fiber of the living matrix, both outside and inside of the cells and nuclei, is surrounded by an organized layer of water that can serve as a separate channel of communication and energy flow." Communication also occurs, he claims, through solid-state biochemistry, crystalline arrays, piezoelectricity and a living tensegrity network; forming a mechanical and vibratory continuum that absorbs healing energies and converts them into acoustic signals. "Each molecule, cell, tissue, and organ has an ideal resonant frequency that coordinates its activities."

Energetic bodywork somehow opens and balances information channels to prevent disease and maintain health. Acupuncture, acupressure, Shiatsu, massage and various forms of structural integration all activate tissue repair processes. It has been found that HRV or Heart Rate Variability (variation in the time interval between heartbeats) relates to emotions. With training, one can achieve a state of internal coherence with a HRV of almost zero. This is a health promoting calm state where you are aware of your electrical body. DNA acts as a resonant antenna to receive and transmit information coded in the heart's electrical rhythms and in the oscillations of the DNA molecules themselves. A sensitive individual can learn to tune in to these phenomena by focusing on any particular body rhythm such as: heart rate, cerebrospinal fluid pulsations or breathing.

Another explanation of the efficacy of microcurrent is through comparison to acupuncture. Many of the effects of acupuncture have been documented in the Journal of the American Medical Association. A "meridian", or energy communication system connecting all parts of the body, has been described by traditional Chinese and Japanese acupuncture. The work of Becker and Nordenstrom in particular recognize the action of subtle electrical currents, via the perineural cells and circulatory system, respectively, in explaining at least part of the meridian phenomenon.

Needle acupuncture is the original microcurrent therapy, as traditional acupuncture needles generate measurable electrical charges when twirled in the skin by a doctor's fingers, and needles left "in situ" tend to drain off excess electric charge from tense or inflamed tissue. Modern microcurrent therapy offers a simplified and non-hazardous method for practitioners to offer the benefits of ancient acupuncture techniques to their patients.

The current practice of medicine is based upon the Newtonian model of reality. This model is primarily a viewpoint which sees the world as an intricate mechanism where doctors conceptualize the body as a type of grand machine, controlled by the brain and peripheral nervous system. A new viewpoint of healing sees matter as an expression of energy having its' basis in the Einsteinian Paradigm and is often referred to as Vibrational Medicine. The Einsteinian model of reality as applied to Vibrational Medicine sees human beings as networks of complex energy fields that interface with cellular systems. Vibrational medicine utilizes and incorporates various forms of energy, such as electrical energy, to positively affect those energetic systems that are out of balance due to disease. The goal is to restore homeostasis and cellular equilibrium by rebalancing the energy fields and energetic dynamics of the organism. The recognition that all matter is energy forms the foundation for understanding how humans can be considered dynamic energetic systems. Through his famous equation, $E=mc^2$, Albert Einstein proved that energy and matter are dual expressions of the same universal substance.

CHAPTER 5

THE CELLULAR PHYSIOLOGY OF HEALING WITH MICRO-CURRENT

Electrical signals allow information to flow through the nervous system extremely rapidly. It all starts with the formation of an electrochemical gradient. The active transport of ions across the cell membrane causes an electrical gradient to build up across this membrane. The number of positively charged ions outside the cell is usually greater than the number of positively charged ions inside the cell. This results in a relatively negative charge on the inside of the membrane, and a positive charge on the outside. This difference in charge causes a voltage to exist across the membrane. Voltage is the electrical potential energy that is caused by a separation of opposite charges, in this case across the cell membrane. The voltage across a membrane is also referred to as the membrane potential. Membrane potential is necessary for the conduction of electrical impulses along nerve cells. The membrane potential of a cell at rest is known as its resting potential. A non-excited nerve cell is an example of a cell at rest.

Since, in the normal healthy state, there are less positive ions inside the cell, the inside of the cell is negative relative to outside the cell. This resulting membrane potential favors the movement of positively charged ions into the cell, and the movement of negative ions out of the cell. So, there are two forces that drive the diffusion (exchange) of ions across the cell's plasma membrane; a chemical force (the ions' concentration gradient), and an electrical force (the effect of the membrane potential on the ions' movement). These two forces working together are called an electrochemical gradient, which determines the direction an ion moves by diffusion or active transport across a membrane.

Electrical resistance of tissue with pathology or disease is often higher than that of the immediately surrounding area, which is either normal or less pathological. Regeneration is a series of electrochemical reactions, where electricity, in miniscule quantities, is needed by the cells to provide energy to fuel the regenerative process. The tissue in the area of pathological involvement needs energy in the form of electricity. The patients' body contains more than a sufficient quantity of energy to produce the desired effect. Unfortunately, the electrical resistance in the area of involvement is so high that the body's energy flow will not enter the area because the primary laws of physics require that energy travel along the path of least resistance. As a result, the electrical energy traveling in the body will circumvent the area of pathology. It will always take the path of least resistance, which is around, rather than through, the area of involvement. To resolve this, we must enable the energy to pass into the area of pathology while still obeying these laws. We can do this by increasing the body's ability to actually produce and store energy in the area of involvement.

This is done, by charging the tissue in a manner similar to a battery. Tissue cells, like battery cells, have the ability to hold an electrical charge. The greater the charge on the cell, the less resistant it is to the flow of electrical energy. As the cell charge increases, the molecular kinetic energy in the cell increases. The electro-vibratory rate (EVR) of the cell's molecular structure must increase with the increased kinetic energy (energy of movement).

An increased EVR will be coupled in direct proportion with an increased electro-conductivity (decreased electrical resistance). While functioning as a battery, the charged cell provides some of the energy which is involved in the energy flow equation. In other words, the addition of electrical energy to an area of pathology increases the electrical conductivity of the area and hence allows the body's own energy to enter the area and affect the tissue.

The term for the quantity of charge that a cell can maintain is "capacitance." As the general health of the cell improves, the capacitance increases. In other words, the cell has the capacity to hold a greater charge of energy. Biologically, the capacitance of the cell is directly proportional to the concentration of Adenosine Triphosphate (ATP) in the cell and ranges from about .1 to 3 microfarads. ATP is at least partially responsible for binding electrons, which cumulatively represent the electrical charge and usable energy of the cell. Areas of the body, which manifest pain, are often deficient in ATP. It follows then, that the electrical energy of these areas must be below standard because the body's electrical flow cannot penetrate the resistance.

ATP concentration serves a direct vital function in the active transport mechanism known as the Sodium pump. Active transport means that this system, which is directly responsible for the transmembrane movement of sodium, potassium, calcium, metabolic .waste and metabolites, requires large amounts of energy to move vital ions in and out of the cell. Metabolic waste builds up in toxic concentrations when a cell is not respiring and metabolizing properly.

The energy which is released when ATP breaks down, fuels the reactions which establish balanced membrane potential gradients and which bring vital metabolites into the cell in exchange for metabolic wastes which are dumped into the general circulation to be detoxified and excreted. What we have when the sodium pump is not functioning is a hypo-polarized, toxic, starving cell.

Re-establishment of the sodium pump occurs when the increase in intracellular current increases mitochondrial function. The increased EVR of the mitochondria enhances the production of ATP in the cytoplasm. The ATP provides the fuel for the transmigration of metabolites and metabolic waste across the cell membrane as well as the reestablishment of cellular bio-electronic ionic concentration gradients.

What this means is that the cell membrane potential, normally .85mv in healthy tissue, is reestablished, while levels of intracellular metabolic waste (ie; lactic acid) are reduced and fresh concentrations of usable cellular metabolites are introduced into the exhausted cell. At this point the cell can enter its regenerative phase, pain levels are noticeably reduced and tissue regeneration functions are reestablished.

The investigations of living cells based on electrical concepts and using electrical techniques have been amazingly successful. For over a half-century, the membranes of cells have been discovered and described. The electrical parameters of cellular metabolism are well known facts and include: resting potential, capacitance, resistance, conductance, impedance, polarization capacity, current density, inductive reactance and electrical phase angle, to name a few.

According to Biophysicist Mark Biedebach, if the integrity of the epidermal tissue is broken by a wound, there will be a net flow of ionic current through the low resistance pathway of the injured cells and the fluid exudate which lines the wound. Therefore, it is tempting to hypothesize that the ionic current flow pattern between normal and insulted tissue plays an important role in stimulating plasma membrane repair processes, essential to the restoration of that tissue to a normal functional state. It follows logically that the rates at which these processes occur may be accelerated by judicious imposition of an electric current from an outside source.

Cellular physiologists are now recognizing that stimuli which activate most energy-requiring processes within cells do so via an increase in intracellular calcium. An increase in intracellular calcium following membrane depolarization occurs because: (1) voltage sensitive Calcium channels allow extra-cellular Calcium to enter (2) current entering the cell can cause Calcium release from cellular organelles.

Biedebach suggests that the best way to alleviate pain and inflammation would be to accelerate the rate of repair of the damaged tissue cell membranes that are responsible for releasing pain-producing substances. Damaged plasma membranes release arachidonic acid, a component of the phospholipid structure of the membrane itself. From this, prostaglandins are synthesized, triggering a cascade of reactions resulting in the release of histamine and bradykinins, which can stimulate pain endings as well as partake in the inflammatory response.

Electrical current that does eventually enter a cell, alters the cell membrane voltage in such a way that it allows an influx of ions, which can turn on and accelerate biochemical processes, essential to cellular repair. If we used only DC current, the intracellular current would flow only through discrete pores or ion-channels, through a low resistance pathway called tight junctions. By using pulsed current, there's an additional pathway for current to enter a cell through membrane capacitance. Current flow through this additional pathway increases the ratio of intracellular to extra-cellular current flow, making the current more effective.

Pulsed current with a rapid voltage rise-time is more effective because: (1) pulsed voltage must rise to its maximum value before membrane capacitance has had time to "Charge up." The time it takes for membrane capacitance to charge up is a fraction of a millisecond. Therefore, it is desirable for the loaded stimulus pulse voltage to rise to its maximum in 50 microseconds or less. (2) Voltage sensitive sodium and calcium channels stay open only (0.5) milliseconds after they have been opened, and they don't re-open for a brief time following closure. The stimulus pulse needs to stay on long enough so that cell membrane capacitance can charge to its maximum value before the pulse turns off. Therefore, duration should last several milliseconds to meet known cellular time constraints. These parameters are appropriately addressed by the Electro-Acuscope and Myopulse technology.

CHAPTER 6

THE SCIENCE BEHIND
THE ACUSCOPE / MYOPULSE
MICRO-CURRENT INSTRUMENTATION

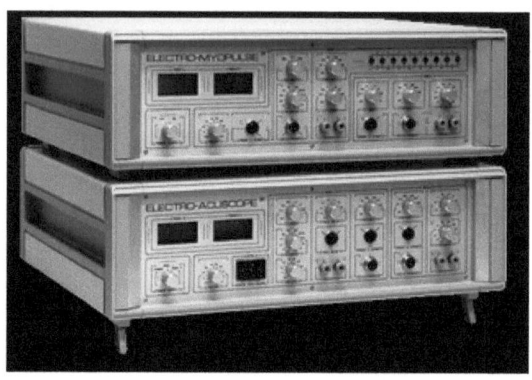

It was in the early 1980's that brought the development of the Electro-Acuscope and Myopulse system; the first in a line of intelligent neural micro-amperage technology. The Acuscope / Myopulse system is a multidimensional analytical microprocessor, constructed electronically to evaluate the transient electrical behavior of the living cell membrane. These; alternating current (AC), microcurrent instruments stimulate tissue repair at the cellular level, rather than muscle contraction.

Physicist Dr. Anthony Nebrenski, an electronic genius who developed missile guidance systems for the Star Wars project also helped develop the EEG and EKG. In 1979, he turned his attention to a revolutionary new healing technology which evolved out of research in electro-acupuncture. His work resulted in the creation of two instruments: the Electro-Acuscope and the Electro-Myopulse.

The heart of the system is an analog to digital conversion processing unit coupled with programmable-array-logic-gates (P.A.L.) technology, whose input-output loop is the key feature, setting it apart from all other electro-therapeutic technologies.

This sophisticated bio-microprocessor arrangement integrates electronics with feedback, allowing for two-way communication between tissue and machine. The result of these components working together provides instantaneous, moment by moment, feedback-assisted computer-modulated electronic pulse trains of infinite variation to induce bio-electronic harmony in disrupted tissue.

Utilizing proprietary carrier wave and cybernetic loop technology, the instrument gathers tissue impedance information and in turn provides a gentle current with waveform control that *whispers* electronic information to the tissues, providing energy medicine that accelerates the body's own natural healing abilities

In other words, biofeedback mechanisms combined with solid state circuitry (microprocessors with preprogrammed memory of tissue equilibrium values) enables the body to automatically control the necessary treatment parameters required for healing by regulating output voltage levels from the instrument based on amplified and filtered input of biological events (those events occurring in the tissues being addressed).

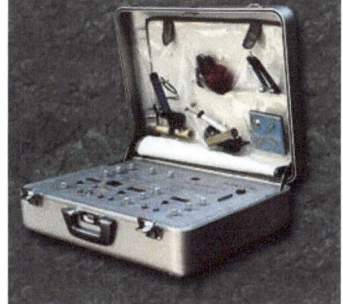

All biological events observed within the input-output loop is; defined in accordance with the master program - a neural network thermodynamic model which performs high-speed formulations. This technology communicates with the body by monitoring and transmitting **corrective treatments** based on existing conductivity and other electromagnetic measures. This is accomplished by the design of equilibrium principles, stored in a unique circuit microchip and other discrete components. These complex units acquire the actual value of the treatment area through the input electrodes and then compare them to the desired value. If there is any difference between the actual tissue value and the preset equilibrium principles, a digital signal is sent out to another component to process and initiate appropriate responses to achieve a physiological **steady state** that promotes normal cell membrane resting tension. By normalizing cell membrane resting tension, other cellular dependent electrical characteristics such as capacitance, polarity, resistance and ph can also be normalized.

Using *Fourier Transform Analysis*, a high speed computerized algorithm, it is possible to determine numerous parameters from current and voltage waveforms. The Acuscope and Myopulse; samples a series of data values from the waveforms of the stimulus current as well as the voltage between the electrodes. Analog-to-digital conversion circuitry continuously computes magnitude and phase angle of the impedance characteristics over a range of frequencies. If these characteristics are different than those found in normal tissue, or if changes occur during stimulation, the digital program then adjusts the delivery of pulses and current to deliver optimal intracellular current to stimulate cellular repair processes in a most effective and efficient way.

If adjustments are not made in magnitude and waveform, there is no assurance that the current, which flows intracellularly is maintained at optimal value during treatment. This makes monitoring of the impedance values (or tissue conductance) highly desirable and necessary in order to promote cellular repair and the advantage of using computer-assisted circuitry (such as that found in the Electro-Acuscope and Myopulse) to regulate and continually adjust the magnitude and / or wave-shape of the stimulus pulses. These instruments have also been calibrated as distinct devices for use in the Veterinarian as well as the cosmetic industries.

The Acuscope uses frequency specific microcurrent via specialized probes over foot reflexology zones, Odonton reflex points over the gums and can deliver Nogier resonance frequencies to treat acupoints on the ear without using needles. These frequencies can be manipulated by the operator as the need arises. Similar to reflexology, in which treatment is administered through the foot, auriculotherapy operates on the concept that the entire body and all its organs can be identified at different points on the ear. The somatotopology of the body is also represented in the gums, the scalp and other reflex zones. Although Auriculotherapy is traditionally practiced with acupuncture needles, the Electro Acuscope uses a noninvasive hand held probe with a special calibrated spring loaded tip to correctly interface with the acupoints on the ear. When used for auricular therapy, pre-prescribed protocols can be used or the practitioner can take a radial pulse during the treatment. The increase or decrease in radial pulse amplitude, called the vascular autonomic signal (VAS), is used as an indicator for the progression of treatment. This mode of treatment requires considerable training.

Assessment of information after the point is located is done internally by the circuitry and does not require interpretation by the operator. However, I have personally found it helpful to understand the gain spectrum function of the instrument, which has allowed me to quickly zero in on the appropriate points that needed treatment, both with the auricular and foot reflexology probes. Higher than normal resistance at a specific acupoint indicates irritation or inflammation in the corresponding organ, while lower than normal resistance at the acupoint is indicative of degeneration or fatigue. These measures can be seen and heard on the meters of the acuscope. Although this information might be of some benefit to the practitioner, the FDA does not allow a device to assess, giving diagnostic information and then treat the point without practitioner intervention. (Medical instruments do not have a license to practice medicine). After a sensitive and appropriate point is assessed, the therapeutic component can be applied by the practitioner. Humans cannot work as fast as an electronic device. Until the FDA adjusts its guidelines for the new era of high speed computers, the Acuscope simply performs the task that is needed without providing any kind of definitive diagnostic information to the operator.

I did have one miraculous case of a fellow practitioner that complained of extended chronic hearing loss on one side of her body. I proceeded to treat the ear point on the same sided foot and during treatment she reported a: "popping sound," followed by a return of her hearing. It happened so fast, it was hard to believe.

In Summary: The Electro-Acuscope and Myopulse technologies use a combination of assessment and treatment protocols, working under the assumption that all biological processes are bio-electromagnetic and can be recognized by a distinctive, complex waveform. A smooth wave indicates health, and higher or lower wave deviations indicate disease. The Electro Acuscope collects electromagnetic signals directly from acupoints or other areas that are specifically targeted, manipulates and adjusts any aberrant waveforms to create normal waves, and then feeds these corrected waves of energy back into the patient through the same treatment areas or points. These devices are truly a natural therapy as they use specific wave information from the patient without introducing artificial or synthesized wave forms such as "current tens units or zapper devises." The carrier waves that transfer such information from the tissue for assessment is truly innovative since the bio-information that is sought is below the Niquist noise levels of electronic instruments or thermal noise in electronic circuits (the electronic *noise* generated by the thermal agitation of the charge carriers, usually electrons.

During treatment, there is little or no sensation because micro-current energy is similar to the energy inside the body. Micro-currents are one-millionth the strength of household current. They are compatible with the body's bioelectrical communication system and support the self-healing feedback mechanism already present at the cellular level. The effects' of micro-currents on the healing process has been documented in the scientific literature for many years.

When this energy is introduced into the cells, circulation, lymphatic drainage, waste product removal and cellular metabolism improve. The flow of other forms of biological energy similar to chi or vital force is accelerated. Acidic waste products are flushed from the tissues and the body's healing powers are accentuated. This results in an accelerated healing response at the cellular level, leading to reduction of pain and improved function.

Since its success in treating injuries at the 1984 Olympic Games in Los Angeles, the Acuscope and Myopulse have been used extensively to treat Olympic, collegiate and professional athletes, as well as thousands of patients in the arena of pain and rehabilitative medicine. Acuscope and Myopulse treatment is completely safe and may be the only treatment necessary for a relatively recent injury. In older conditions, additional procedures such as manual muscle therapy, manipulative therapy and therapeutic exercises are usually helpful in achieving the best overall recovery.

The Electro-Acuscope is designed to scan and treat many types of pain. It is an FDA classified Biofeedback instrument. The central and autonomic nervous systems of your body are balanced by this technology without needles or discomfort.

The Acuscope system is currently being used by professional athletic teams, sports medicine practices, hospitals and thousands of private physicians and therapists in every field of medicine. The Acuscope is very effective with animals and is being used extensively in veterinary as well as human medicine.

According to widespread publicity, many outstanding athletes have been significantly helped by Electro-Acuscope treatment; several who received Acuscope treatments for pain and injury won gold medals during various Olympic Games.

Each Acuscope treatment can last anywhere from 15 to 40 minutes. The relief is cumulative; in other words, the relief will last longer and longer with each additional treatment. The goal, of course, is permanent relief. After an initial series of 3-5 treatments, possibly a few more, many people have permanent pain relief and never need another Electro-Acuscope treatment for the same condition. For some, the relief is more temporary and booster treatments may be needed as often as weekly, monthly, or as seldom as once or twice a year. Frequency and duration of treatment is tailored to meet individual needs, which is dependent on numerous variables.

Acuscope treatments are usually painless. A small percentage of patients feel a tiny pulse, or just a slight stinging like tiny needles lightly pricking the skin. Have no fear, if there is any discomfort whatsoever, simply mention it during treatment and your doctor or therapist will adjust the settings to your comfort. It is not best for you to just "grin and bear it." During treatment, most patients feel nothing except relief and report only the sensations of general relaxation, warmth or a comfortable tingling in the area being treated.

The probes or electrodes are typically moistened utilizing a proprietary transmission gel, after which the electrodes are then applied to the surface of the skin. Some patients with swelling and extreme sensitivity to touch may experience some discomfort from the pressure of the probes, which can easily be modified to comfort.

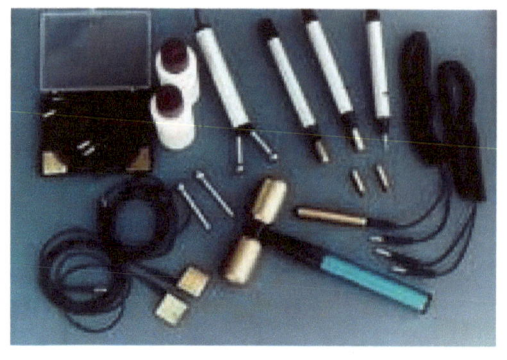

Most patients, however, feel only a gently or firm pressure at the points of contact, or the massaging effect of some of the larger, rounded brass electrodes. Contact pads may be taped in place to provide extended stimulation to a specific area in need of prolonged treatment. Your hands, feet or other surfaces may be placed in contact with the large brass plates; or you may be treated with a headband or ear clip set to produce overall body relief or relaxation. Whichever attachment is used with the Electro-Acuscope, the experience of treatment is generally quite comfortable, most often even enjoyable.

There are no true side-effects; that is, there are no long-term side-effects. Some temporary discomfort may be experienced after the treatment. The possibilities include headache, nausea, and increased pain. Fortunately, these side-effects are rare and usually occur, if at all, following the first one to three treatments only. Any change, including temporary increased discomfort, is a good sign. It shows change is going on in the body; almost anyone who feels some increase in pain immediately or soon after the first treatment has a very good long-term pain relief prognosis. Often you will feel the results during or within several hours after the first or second treatment. A single, thirty-minute treatment is often followed by hours or even days of relief. Occasionally the relief from a single treatment is permanent. Sometimes three or four treatments are necessary before changes begin to take place. In some cases it may take more.

Considerable training is required before using this device. There are prescribe protocols for this treatment and many conditions respond favorably with this technique.

Therapeutic applications include addictions, dyslexia, pain control (acute or chronic pain, back pain, and pain from trauma), tinnitus, Parkinsonian tremors and joint pain of Rhematoid arthritis. It would be contraindicated to use an Electro Acuscope to treat a life threatening condition such as renal insufficiency and heart disease.

The Acusope can be used for point massage and method is popular as a treatment in sports medicine, treating musculoskeletal injuries, such as lumbosacral sprains, shoulder strains, whiplash, trauma, temporomandibular joint pain, bursitis, carpal tunnel syndrome and muscle spasms. It's also used for arthritis, bruises, herpes zoster infections, local skin infections and skin ulcerations, chronic fatigue syndrome, migraines, neuralgia, surgical incisions, and palliative care of a ruptured disk in patients unwilling or unable to undergo surgery. It is particularly helpful in reducing post-surgical pain and inflammatory complications such as excess scarring.

When used to support Chiropractic or Osteopathic spinal manipulation it helps relax the tissue before the adjustment to make the manipulative procedure as gentle and as painless as possible. It also improves the healing of the joint and surrounding tissue so fewer treatments are necessary to control pain or to stabilize joint subluxation reduction.

The Acuscope can correctly identify and discriminate chronic degenerative conditions vs. acute inflammatory conditions and properly program the treatment without guess work by the instruments operator. This is particularly important when doing meridian or reflex point therapy on acupuncture points since the Acuscope properly applies tonification or sedation to the reflex point without guess work and without puncturing the tissue with needles.

The Electro Acuscope significantly reduces pain in chronic as well as acute pain conditions. It helps restore circulation thereby bringing nutrition and oxygen to damaged and scarred tissue. Therefore it helps to reduce scar tissue complications of injury or surgery. Controlled studies have demonstrated the benefits of bioelectrical acupuncture to treat postoperative pain, chemotherapy-induced illness, and renal colic and to induce contractions in post-term pregnancy.

There are many indications for Electro Acuscope and Myopulse treament: Inflammatory conditions: Tendinitis, bursitis, Degenerative arthritis, Acute inflammatory arthritis such as rheumatoid arthritis, Tennis elbow, Carpal tunnel syndrome. Chronic pain conditions such as: Fibromyalgia, Reflex sympathetic dystrophy, Neuralgia (nerve pain), radiating pain in arms or legs, headache pain and myalgias (muscle pain). Also for fibromyalgia, facial pain associated with TMJ syndrome, trigger point/myofascial pain syndromes (overload contracture reflexes). For acute injuries: sprains (torn or overstretched ligaments), strains (torn or overstretched muscles), post-surgical pain and inflammation such as post joint replacement or arthroscopic surgery and fractures. Wound Healing: Dicubitus ulcers and Diabetic venous stasis ulcers.

CHAPTER 7

Fourier Transform: How the Acuscope Technology Actually Works

One of the Fundamental Secrets of the Universe: All waveforms, no matter what you scribble or observe in the universe, are actually just the sum of different frequencies.

The Fourier Transform decomposes a waveform - basically any real world waveform, into a sinusoid or mathematical curve that is. The Fourier Transform gives us another way to represent a waveform. As an example, let's break down the waveform in Figure 1 into its 'building blocks' (or constituent frequencies).

The first component is a sinusoidal wave with period T=6.28 and amplitude 0.3, as shown in Figure 1.

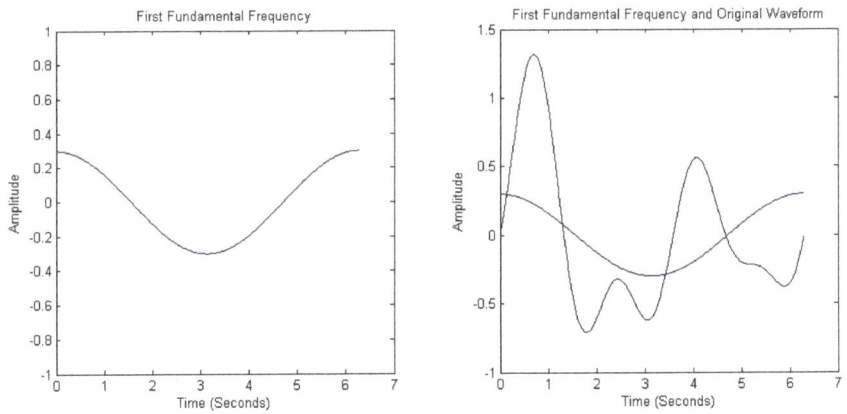

Figure 1. First fundamental frequency (left) and original waveform (right) compared.

The second frequency will have a period half as long as the first (twice the frequency). The second component is shown on the left in Figure 2, along with the sum of the first two frequencies compared to the original waveform.

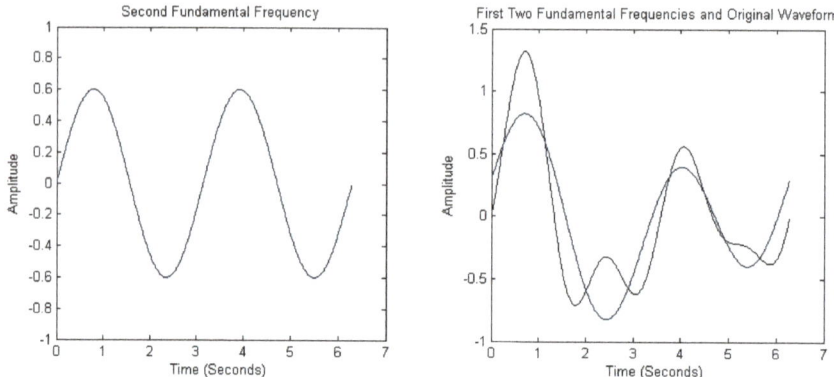

Figure 2. Second fundamental frequency (left) and original waveform compared with the first two frequency components.

We see that the sum of the first two frequencies is starting to look like the original waveform. The third frequency component is 3 times the frequency as the first. The sum of the first three components are illustrated in Figure 3.

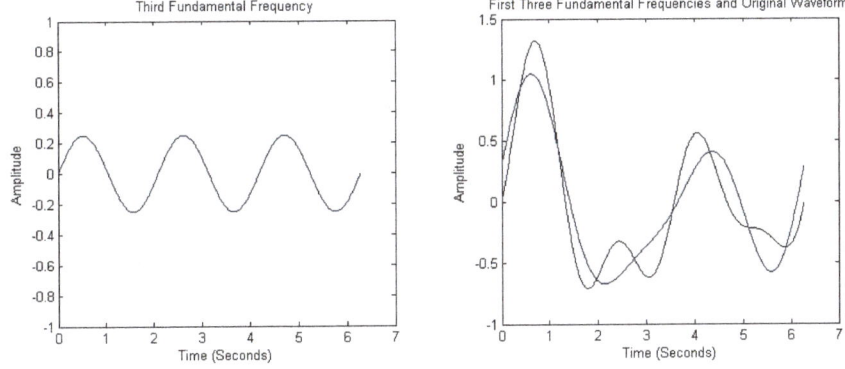

Figure 3. Third fundamental frequency (left) and original waveform compared with the first three frequency components.

Finally, adding in the fourth frequency component, we get the original waveform, shown in Figure 4.

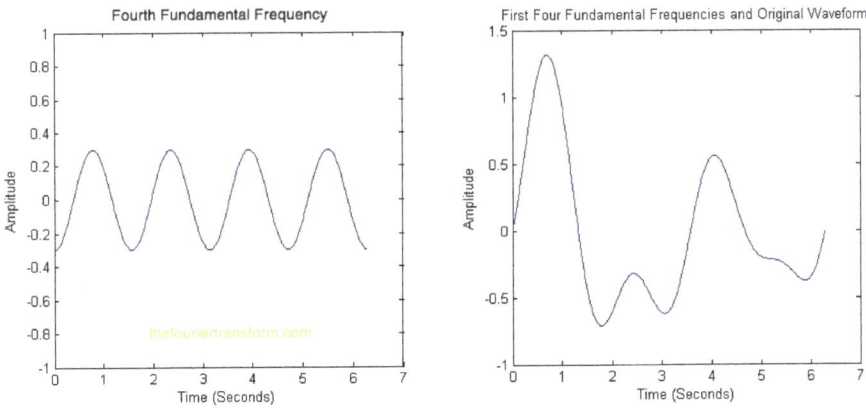

Figure 4. Fourth fundamental frequency (left) and original waveform compared with the first four frequency components

While this seems made up, it is true for all waveforms. This goes for TV signals, cell phone signals and sound waves that travel when you speak. In general, waveforms are not made up of a discrete number of frequencies, but rather a continuous range of frequencies.

The Fourier Transform is the mathematical tool that shows us how to deconstruct the waveform into its sinusoidal components. This has a multitude of applications, aides in the understanding of the universe, and just makes life much easier for the practicing engineer or scientist.

The Fourier transform decomposes a function of time (a *signal*) into the frequencies that make it up, similar to how a musical chord can be expressed as the amplitude (or loudness) of its constituent notes.

Here's a plain-English metaphor:

- **What does the Fourier Transform do?** Given a smoothie, it finds the recipe.
- **How?** Run the smoothie through filters to extract each ingredient.
- **How do we get the smoothie back?** Blend the ingredients.

Here's the "math English" version: The Fourier Transform takes a time-based pattern, measures every possible cycle, and returns the overall "cycle recipe" (the strength, offset, & rotation speed for every cycle that was found).

From Smoothie to Recipe.

The Fourier Transform changes our perspective from *what did I see?* Into; *how was it made?* In other words: given a smoothie, let's find the recipe. Why? Well, recipes are great descriptions of drinks. You wouldn't share a drop-by-drop analysis; you'd say "I had an orange/banana smoothie". A recipe is more easily categorized, compared, and modified than the object itself. So... given a smoothie, how do we find the recipe?

Smoothie to Recipe

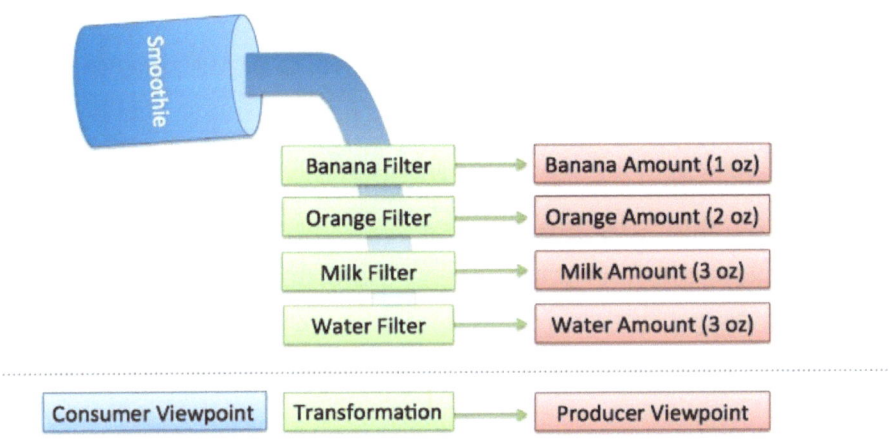

- Pour through the "banana" filter. 1 oz of bananas are extracted.
- Pour through the "orange" filter. 2 oz of oranges.
- Pour through the "milk" filter. 3 oz of milk.
- Pour through the "water" filter. 3 oz of water.

We can reverse-engineer the recipe by filtering each ingredient. The catch?

- **Filters must be independent**. The banana filter needs to capture bananas, and nothing else. Adding more oranges should never affect the banana reading.
- **Filters must be complete**. We won't get the real recipe if we leave out a filter
- **Ingredients must be combine-able**. Smoothies can be separated and re-combined without issue (A cookie? Not so much. Who wants crumbs?). The ingredients, when separated and combined in any order, must produce the same result.

The Fourier Transform finds the recipe for a signal, like our smoothie process:

- Start with a time-based signal
- Apply filters to measure each possible " ingredient"
- Collect the full recipe, listing the amount of each "ingredient"

If earthquake patterns can be separated into ingredients, vibrations of different speeds & strengths, buildings can be designed to avoid interacting with the strongest ones. If sound waves can be separated into ingredients (bass and treble frequencies), we can boost the parts we care about, and hide the ones we don't. The crackle of random noise can be removed, such as during signal to noise ratio on the radio.

If computer data can be represented with oscillating patterns, perhaps the least-important ones can be ignored. These compression techniques are used to reduce data size for storage, handling, and for transmitting content, drastically shrinking file sizes (and why JPEG and MP3 files are much smaller than raw .bmp or .wav files). If a radio wave is our signal, we can use filters to listen to a particular channel.

How do we split sound into frequencies? our ears do it by mechanical means, mathematicians do it using Fourier transforms and computers by Fast Fourier Transforms.

CHAPTER 8

BRADSHAW GETS NEW HOPE
FROM THE SCOPE

Bradshaw Gets New Hope from the 'Scope': The Miracle Machine recharged the arm of Terry Bradshaw, who juiced up the Steelers' playoff prospects.

By Jill Lieber

Art Rooney, the 82-year-old owner of the Pittsburgh Steelers, toddled into the training room at Three Rivers Stadium recently to see for himself what all the commotion was about. At one end of the room sat an 18X12X4-inch metal box with a pencil-like device dangling from it on a cord. The box was blinking and beeping, doing all sorts of space-age stuff.

What do we have here?" Rooney said, poking his way through a crowd of players. "Somebody from the circus? "

"No, Boss," replied Terry Bradshaw, the Steeler quarterback who missed Pittsburgh's first 14 games this season with an ailing throwing arm, "it's the Miracle Machine."

"Hmmm..... Miracle Machine?" Rooney said with a laugh. "Let me try." He held out his arthritic right hand. Terry Eberhardt, a physical therapist from Shreveport, La., ran the "pencil" over Rooney's hand. The pain vanished. Rooney stared at his hand.... and stared.... and stared. He jumped up and bounced down the hall, stopping everybody he saw. "Look at this!" he exclaimed, making a fist for the first time in almost two years.

"Isn't it amazing?" Bradshaw said. "I just love this thing!"

And no wonder. The Miracle Machine, a.k.a. Acuscope, has given the 35 year-old Bradshaw new life, and in the process it has given a big boost, to the Steelers' playoff prospects.

A month ago Bradshaw's right arm was so sore from off-season elbow surgery and a strained triceps that it was virtually useless. After having used that arm to throw for 27,912 yards and 210 touchdowns in his 14-year NFL career, Bradshaw had become almost completely a lefthander. "Just squeezing something brought him to his knees in pain," Eberhardt says. But on Nov. 19, Bradshaw began to undergoing daily treatments on the Acuscope system and, well... Do you believe in miracles?

Last Saturday at Shea Stadium, Bionic Bradshaw took the field with his Miracle Machine Arm and picked apart the New York Jets. He hadn't taken a snap from center in an NFL game since Jan uary 9th, but on the Steelers' second series, with Jet Defensive End Mark Gastineau dancing in his face, Bradshaw tossed a 17-yard touchdown pass to Greg Garrity. He came back early in the second quarter to hit Calvin Sweeney over the middle with a 10-yard scoring throw for a 14-0 lead. "I was nervous," Bradshaw said afterward, "but once I got on the field it was like a duck taking to water."

After his second touchdown pass, Bradshaw had to leave the game. He'd bruised his right elbow, having hit it on a Jet's helmet on one play and fallen on it on another. He'd completed five of eight passes for 77 yards, and later, in the locker room, he vowed he'd be back for the playoffs.

Going into the game against New York, Pittsburgh badly needed to be energized. It had lost three straight after a 9-2 start, and in those three defeats, Bradshaw's backup, Cliff Stoudt, had been inept, completing only 30 of 74 passes (40.5%) for 339 yards, with six interceptions and just two TDs.

"Terry sent waves of confidence through the entire team," Steeler Coach Chuck Noll said. Indeed, Pittsburgh beat the Jets easily, 34-7, and that win, coupled with Cleveland's 34-27 loss to Houston on Sunday, gave the Steelers the AFC Central title. All of which meant Pittsburg could rest Bradshaw until its first playoff game, on New Year's Eve or New Year's Day.

There were times during the last eight months when Bradshaw didn't know what the next week - or even the next day - would bring. He'd strained his elbow severely in the '82 training camp and got through last season on weekly cortisone shots. Even before last season, a Shreveport orthopedic surgeon, Dr. Bill Bundrick, had diagnosed the ailment as "reverse tennis elbow" – micro-tears of the flexor pronator muscle, which is located over the inside of the elbow - and on March 3rd of this year he removed the damaged tissue and reattached the muscle. Bradshaw was told not to throw until July. But by Pittsburgh's May minicamp Bradshaw was feeling like his old self. He began throwing and tore more tissue in his elbow, which ballooned to the size of a softball. Bundrick told Bradshaw not to even think of playing before September. "I felt like scolding him," the doctor says. "But he can't help it. He's Terry Bradshaw."

By September the swelling and pain hadn't subsided, so the Steelers sent Bradshaw to physical therapists in Pittsburgh. He subsequently made a trip to Shreveport to see

Bundrick and while there tested a new gadget the doctor had just bought - the Acuscope, which simulates the effects of acupuncture by increasing the electrical activity of cells, thereby promoting healing. Bradshaw used it just once and was a changed man. He began lobbing balls 30 to 40 yards. By late October he was itching to play. He threw and he threw and he threw - up to three hours and 1,500 balls a day. Soon he had a strained triceps. "It was a totally different injury," Bundrick says; "One from sheer overuse."

Out of frustration, Bradshaw and Noll began exchanging words in the newspapers. Bradshaw charged that Noll didn't care about him; Noll suggested that perhaps Bradshaw was ready for his "life's work," that maybe he ought to retire.

Bradshaw fled to Shreveport and the Acuscope. After one treatment he had 60% relief from the pain and swelling of the strained triceps; the next day, he had 80% relief. Ten days later, on the Monday following Thanksgiving, Bradshaw went back to Pittsburgh, this time with the Acuscope following close behind. He promised that a miracle had been performed. Noll was skeptical. But after seeing Bradshaw work out, Noll realized he had his old quarterback back. "I believe in miracles," he says now.

In the meantime half the Steelers have started using the Acuscope, and Rooney is ready to shell out $7,500 for the team's very own machine.

Sports Illustrated Dec. 19, 1983 Volume 59, No. 26

CHAPTER 9

THE ELECTROSLEEP MODE OF
THE ELECTRO-ACUSCOPE

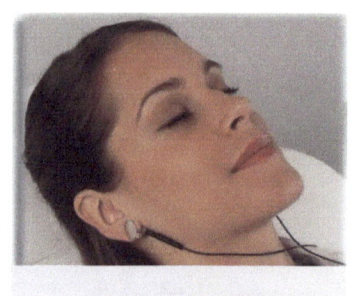

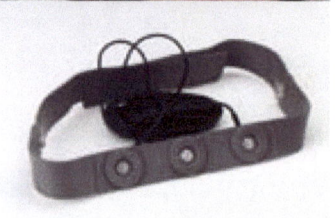

Another ancillary procedure that attention should also be directed to is the Acuscope's capacity in managing and assisting people with stress-related imbalances.

One of the most promising advances in Electro-Medicine today is cranial electrotherapy stimulation or CES. This therapy usually uses less than one milliampere of current directed through the brain for the treatment of anxiety, insomnia and depression; all of which are universal and pervasive in pain patients.

Low intensity electrical stimulation is believed to have originated in the studies of galvanic currents in humans and animals as conducted by Giovanni Aldini, Alessandro Volta and others in the 18th century. Aldini had experimented with galvanic head current as early as 1794 upon himself while also reporting the successful treatment of patients suffering from melancholia using direct low-intensity currents in 1804.

About 100 years after Giovanni Aldini's experiments on medical galvanism, Dr. Louise Robinovitch, a Russian physician, took the use of electricity to the next level. In 1905, Robinovitch thought that electric shocks could restart the hearts of people who died suddenly.

After Robinovitch's initial experiments on animals, she tried it on a woman who did die with those circumstances. She switched the electricity on and off at the same rhythm as the beating heart and soon the woman's heart started beating normally. Robinovitch proceeded to design a machine that could deliver electric currents to patients in an emergency. Today we call this machine a defibrillator. Robinovitch went on to publish "Electric Sleep" in 1905 on the use of electricity for other issues such as electro anesthesia as a substitute for traditional anesthetics. Current interest in Crainal Electric Stimulation or CES was initiated by Robinovitch, who in 1914 made the first claim for electrical treatment of insomnia.

CES is a form of non-invasive brain stimulation that applies a low intensity, pulsed micro-electric current across a person's head (applied to the earlobes or scalp) with the intention of treating a variety of conditions such as anxiety, depression and insomnia. CES has been suggested as a possible treatment for headaches, fibromyalgia, smoking cessation and opiate withdrawal. Electrodes are placed on the ear lobes, maxilla-occipital junction, mastoid processes or temples.

Researchers at several major universities in America and elsewhere along with the Veterans Medical Centers are establishing the analgesic effects of CES for chronic intractable pain such as in spinal cord injuries. The latest cranial electrotherapy stimulation research is showing dramatic improvement in pain throughout the body from such difficult management problems as fibromyalgia, spinal cord injuries, and chronic regional pain syndrome utilizing micro-current applied across the brain.

Despite the long history of CES, its underlying principles and mechanisms are still not clear. CES stimulation of 1 mA (miliampere) has shown to reach the thalamic area of the brain. CES has shown to induce changes in the electroencephalogram, increasing alpha relative power and decreasing relative power in delta and beta frequencies. CES has also been shown to reach cortical and subcortical areas of the brain, in electromagnetic tomography and functional MRI studies.

CES treatments have been found to induce changes in neuro-hormones and neurotransmitters that have been implicated in psychiatric disorders: substantial increases in beta endorphins, adrenocorticotrophic hormones, serotonin; moderate increases in melatonin and norepinephrine, modest or unquantified increases in cholinesterase, gamma-aminobutyric-acid, dehydroepiandrosterone and moderate reductions in cortisol.

CES was initially studied for insomnia and called Electrosleep Therapy; it is also known as cranial-electro stimulation and transcranial electrotherapy. With the invention of the transistor in the 1960's, small, low power and reliable CES devices were developed.

In 1972, a specific form of CES was developed by Dr. Margaret Patterson. The treatment used small pulses of electric current across the head for acute and chronic withdrawal from addictive substances. It was named "NeuroElectric Therapy (NET)." By 1975 several companies in the US and Europe were manufacturing CES devices for public use. During this time, research on CES was quite active and scientific papers were published.

CES is a prescription device, which became available in the United States in 1963 as Electrosleep. The device was grandfathered into modern FDA regulation in 1976 as a Class III device under the Medical Device Amendments Act of 1976, when the name was changed to Cranial Electrotherapy Stimulation. Most studies to date have shown CES as a reliable method to reduce anxiety and improve cognition in recovering alcoholics. Additional studies have shown CES to be an effective tool in reducing anxiety and improving IQ.

Due to the rise of pharmaceutical treatments for depression, anxiety and insomnia, such as Prozac in the 1980s and Ambien in the 1990s, CES was not a well-known treatment for doctors and patients. During the mid-2000s, the combination of pharmaceutical brands becoming generic and internet advertising caused CES devices to gain popularity. In 2011, the devices received more media attention from the *Wall Street Journal*.

By placing special electrodes on the ear lobes or the frontal bone of the head, CES, when set at the appropriate frequencies, will induce a relaxed concentration in the client within 20 to 30 minutes. This procedure, also known as "Electro-Sleep," or "cranial electric stimulation" has been applied successfully by medical specialists ranging from dentists to psychiatrists. In addition to enhancing brainwave entrainment, CES increases neurotransmitter production. These neurotransmitters are necessary for information processing, memory, energy level and physical well-being. When our neurotransmitters and endorphins are not produced to necessary levels, it may lead to destructive behaviors and/or the abuse of substances as a substitute for that "natural high."

This procedure is recommended to reduce mental fatigue, enhance autonomic stability, improve concentration, and, as a general procedure, to prepare the patient for treatment, including surgery. This procedure can also be helpful with hyperactive children, depression/manic depression, insomnia, anxiety, headache, migraines, visual disturbances and head trauma.

Other research investigations demonstrate the promise of electro-sleep in other lifestyle stress-related areas such as obesity, addiction, compulsion, alcohol and drug detox, mood/food, etc. Unlike drug therapy, there is no dependency, adverse side effects, and benefits are sustained for progressively longer periods of time permitting increased conditioning to behavior modification methods.

The electro-sleep phenomenon occurs when a relaxed state is induced by the transcranial application of low intensity current. Actually, the word "electro-sleep" is misleading in that patients are not forced into sleep; but rather guided into a relaxed, conscious state.

Most of the research and scientific investigations on electro-sleep have been conducted in the Soviet Union for the past few decades. There has been very limited research conducted here in the United States. A great deal of this hesitancy is probably due to the traditional mistrust of the use of electrical devices in clinical psychiatry. A few studies conducted at certain universities have produced interesting results.

Groups of patients with chronic anxiety, depression, and nocturnal insomnia were selected on the basis that they have had little or no positive response to orthodox methods of treatment. These patients had all utilized various types of sleeping medications for long periods of time with poor results. The use of electro-sleep with these same patients, however, showed significant improvements in their conditions. The most marked result was an increase in sleep.

Altering your Brainwaves:
The Secret to Personal Transformation

The short end of the stick is that all inner change or personal transformation happens at a deeper level of consciousness. No matter how brilliant our thoughts and ideas are, they are not sufficient to bring about real change. When it comes down to making powerful and positive shifts in our life, knowledge by itself is superfluous. That means that you can conceptually and rationally grasp the secrets of the universe but you can only put them into practice by integrating them into your totality of self.

The idea of course is nothing new. Ancient spiritual practices such as meditation and Yoga or modern practices such as hypnosis and neuro linguistic programming (NLP) have at their core the common goal of accessing deeper levels of consciousness and using those states to reprogram the mind. Deep healing, intuition, tapping into your amazing source of creativity and changing counterproductive beliefs are some of the things that are easily achievable through tuning into your deeper states of mind.

Psychology talks about the notion of the subconscious and unconscious as facets of our psyche that lie beneath the threshold of conscious thought and reasoning. Ultimately these are just labels to parts of our self we know very little of.

Modern research in neuroscience has been discovering facts that merge with or complement ancient knowledge and wisdom. One interesting area of research is that of brainwaves and how they correlate to states of mind and levels of consciousness. Brain waves are practically; waves that are produced by the synchronized electrical pulses when clusters of brain neurons are communicating with each other.

Brainwaves, as they are received by an electrode on the surface of the scalp, are the sum of electro-chemical language passing through a very large group of nerves (hundreds of millions). This sum generates two primary characteristics: Amplitude and Frequency. Amplitude is measured in microvolts - frequency is measured in Hertz (Hz) or cycles per second. These basic characteristics are believed to be determined by the degree of synchronized activity inherent in the group of brain cells being monitored. When this activity is synchronized, the amplitude is higher and the frequency is lower. Brainwaves have been categorized into four basic levels on the basis of frequency: DELTA: 0.1 to 3.5 Hz, THETA: 3.5 to 7.5 Hz, ALPHA: 7.5 to 14 Hz, and BETA: 14 to 30 Hz.

BETA spectrum waves are dominant in our normal waking consciousness when attention is directed to cognitive tasks and the outside world. It is connected to problem solving, decision making, complex thinking and even anxiety and excitement.

Beta dominated brain states are very energy intensive and represent relatively unsynchronized activity. This activity appears to be chaotic, rapidly changing in frequency and amplitude. It is associated with normal, outward awareness, for example; taking in, evaluation, and filing away of various forms of information received through the senses. It is usually the state when an individual experiences anger, hunger, anxiety, tension and surprise.

The DELTA (0.1 to 3.5 Hz) is opposite to BETA and would be the result of high synchronization. Delta waves are the slowest and loudest waves of the spectrum. They promote healing and regenerative processes. Its slow rate of change is associated with relatively unconscious states such as deep meditation and dreamless sleep.

The ALPHA (7.5 to 14 Hz) spectrum is usually produced as rhythms of steady frequency and amplitude. These waves are emitted when you are in a relaxed and calm state and when you are anchored in the present moment. This state aids learning and mind/body integration. It is associated primarily with pleasant inward awareness, a non-drowsy but relaxed state; a tranquil state of mind. Outside stimulation usually interrupts this alpha rhythm.

The THETA (3.5 to 7.5 Hz) level is associated with an access to unconscious material, drowsiness, fantasy, imagery, dreaming recall, problem solving, inspiration, and creativity. Theta waves occur when we are drifting off in sleep and also present in deep meditation. Theta waves usually accompany intuition and vivid imagery. This state facilitates deep learning and memory and holds information beyond our normal waking consciousness.

Advanced students of Yoga, Zen and other forms of meditation or inner awareness appropriately display an ability to produce enhanced (high amplitude, low frequency) states such as ALPHA and THETA activity.

It is the ALPHA and THETA areas that are increased with the use of the Electro-Acusope. In most cases, after 10 to 30 minutes of treatment, the patient will enter the THETA state. There are a great many benefits to anyone that uses the Electro-Acuscope for this purpose. One 10 to 30 minute treatment with the instrument can replace many hours of rest. It is common for people to need much less rest per night.

Even if you wanted to continue getting as much rest per night as before, patients report that the quality of rest improves. In cases where the sleep cycle is completely disturbed such as trans-continental flight, you can eliminate any jet lag effects with a short session on the Electro-Acuscope, either during flight or upon arrival.

People that work nights and sleep days or have to sleep in a noisy environment, find that they obtain better quality of rest and do not suffer any detrimental effects because of the poor sleeping environment. Executives, students or anyone that works in a high-stress environment obtain great results from the treatments. Many people find that during the day when they feel stressed, they simply find a comfortable reclining chair or bed and take a 10 to 30 minute Electro-Sleep break, which simulates a long nap.

CHAPTER 10

ELECTRO-DERMAL THERAPY

The concept of viewing and treating the body from an energetic perspective has evolved as a result of recent discoveries in quantum physics, even though eastern traditions have included these concepts in their medical system for thousands of years. The meridian system of energy flow is a basic principle within these ancient traditions.

The meridians are a network of energy tracks which extend over the length of the entire body and are considered by some scientists to be the biophysical manifestation of the body's internal organs and the pattern along which the body's bio-energy moves. It is along these meridians where numerous acupuncture points are found.

Modern energetic medicine was strongly influenced by Reinhold Voll, a German physician who, in the 1950's, engineered one of the first devices that measured the electrical charges at acupuncture points. Voll discovered that the electrical parameters of these points were different in healthy and sick people and documented the changes that occurred at those points after medical intervention.

Dr. Voll treated thousands of patients with his electro-diagnostic techniques and discovered additional acupuncture points previously unknown in classical Chinese medicine. Voll correlated many of these points to organ systems and proved that the electrical nature of those points did indeed reflect the health of the organ system to which those points referred.

Voll also discovered that changes would occur in the readings of points when medicinal substances, particularly homeopathic solutions, were given to the patient. This discovery allowed Voll a way to determine the compatibility of those substances when introduced into the patient's energy field. This approach later became known as *Electro-acupuncture According to Voll* or EAV.

The emergence of EAV has resulted in a progressive method that provides information related to the vital state of an individual, and at a sensitivity that allows disturbances to be observed long before the onset of clinical pathology. By detecting energetic imbalances of the body's organs at early stages of dysfunction, EAV can warn the patient of potential future health hazards long before they appear, thus decreasing the possibility of late discovery of a medical condition. Consequently, the results obtained with EAV cannot always be confirmed through clinical methods of examination or laboratory tests since the energetic changes observed with EAV precede the changes in the cells or organs for which evidence can be supported by traditional medical means.

Numerous research articles in professional journals attest to the clinical usefulness of EAV; however, more persuasive documentation is provided by university-based controlled experiments. In 1985, researchers at USC and UCLA demonstrated, in a double-blind study, an 87 percent correlation between EAV measurements of the lung meridian and X-ray diagnosis of patients with lung cancer. Similarly, researchers at the University of Hawaii compared a diabetic population with a control group and demonstrated a 95 to 97.5 percent correlation between EAV and the conventionally confirmed diabetic group.

EAV will not only prove to be of value alongside the diagnostic methods used in conventional medicine, but will likely acquire further recognition as our knowledge increases and as we learn more about the phenomena associated with the energetic information transfer methods by which the human system is regulated. The ability to detect and interpret signals from internal organs at acupuncture points offers exciting medical possibilities. With a greater scientific understanding of the meridian system, this concept could conceivably apply to Western medicine for early detection and identification of health problems and help prevent the progress of many degenerative diseases.

CHAPTER 11

ACUSCOPE: WHAT TO EXPECT

When tissues are diseased or damaged, the normal electrical flow and functioning of the body is disrupted at the cellular level. The cells experience "their power being shut off." Nutrients are unable to flow into the cells and toxins are unable to be released. This results in increased electrical resistance in the problem area, causing the body's electrical currents to flow around the damaged tissue. The Electro-Acuscope has the capacity to drive the current through the resistance and stimulate rapid cellular regeneration.

These state-of-the-art computerized medical instruments are programmed to "read" tissue at a cellular level and compare those readings to optimal or healthy tissue values. The computer then selects the appropriate corrective signal and delivers it to the damaged tissue. The devices continue to read and treat until the tissue electrical flow is normalized.

The Electro-Acuscope is designed to specifically balance neurological tissues, and read all body tissues and systems as well. The Electro-Myopulse specializes in accelerating healing and repair of connective tissues such as bone, muscle, tendon, and ligament. These instruments are bringing phenomenal results in applications as diverse as sports injuries, auto accidents, repetitive motion injuries (carpal tunnel), arthritis, stress reduction and insomnia. The general public now has promising new modes of healing to fight chronic pain, giving us a glimpse of the things to come in this exciting new Century.

After Your Electro-Acuscope Treatment:
A More Detailed Explanation

You have just received the first of a series of Electro-Acuscope treatments. You may have additional questions regarding the instrument, the treatment procedure, and what results to expect. This section is intended to provide a more detailed explanation of this unique electromagnetic instrument and to offer you, and perhaps your family and friends, additional understanding of the type of therapy you are receiving.

May I have an in-depth explanation of how the Electro-Acuscope reduces pain?

The human body is made up of a vast number of cells. In many ways, the cells of the human body act like tiny batteries, storing and releasing energy. Each cell has a measurable electrical charge and therefore there is a constant energy flow maintained between cells throughout the electrical circuitry of the body. When damage or trauma occurs, there is a disruption in the production of electricity and a measurable decrease in the flow of energy through the tissues involved. This condition is generally accompanied by a sensation of pain in the area and usually results in the body's inability to readily repair itself. During treatment, the Electro-Acuscope introduces mild electrical currents into the cells of your body in order to return the tissue to a normal level of electrical activity. This process may be likened to a "jump start" and "putting a charge" on the battery of a car. In this way, the instrument assists the body in accelerating the natural self-healing process.

What do the sound and numbers mean?

Incorporating the most advanced electronic technology, the Electro-Acuscope is capable of detecting subtle electrical blockages and imbalances in the areas of the body. This may be heard as a low- pitched tone from the instrument's biofeedback sound mechanism, and seen as a digital reading which ranges from 1 to 100. When the tissues of the painful area being treated have returned to a highly conductive electrical state, the instrument gives a clear, high pitched tone and the lighted numbers on the instrument face give a read-out consistently over 100.

How much electricity does the Acuscope produce?

The amount of electricity produced by the Acuscope is measured in micro-amps (millionths of an amp), an extremely tiny amount of current in comparison to the amount of electricity flowing from a wall socket. It has been scientifically proven that this level of current produces the most beneficial effect on the body's cells. An Acuscope treatment introduces a gentle, battery generated electrical stimulation in patterns similar to and compatible with that which is constantly flowing through every living person and animal.

Why are the results from an Acuscope treatment cumulative?

By definition, the cumulative effect means that each treatment of a given area will take a shorter amount of time and the pain relief which follows will last longer and longer. Unlike other forms of pain relief, such as therapy with certain drugs, the body does not build up a tolerance to Acuscope treatments. In fact, just the opposite effect occurs. Mild electrical stimulation has been proven to stimulate the cells of the body to produce chemicals which are responsible for cellular energy production and may be thought of as the fuel which allows the cells to begin to repair themselves. As these chemical reactions build up, the body's response to each treatment becomes stronger and stronger and the pain relief lasts longer. With each treatment the tissues are able to repair themselves more completely. In most cases, a series of treatments leads to permanent relief or to a greatly diminished level of pain.

Are there any harmful side-effects and why is it that it may hurt more at some point after treatment?

There are various theories as to why an initial increase in discomfort within 24 hours following the treatment may be experienced. One explanation is that the increased range of motion (sometimes barely noticeable) which often results from an Acuscope treatment will allow you to use muscles, which have been unused for some time. The pain, which can result, is similar to the effect of over-exercising normal muscles and feeling sore afterwards. Therefore, what you may feel is the return of your pain with an additional temporary muscle soreness. Other theories have been postulated as to why it may hurt more initially. If this happens to you, and you are curious, do not be concerned. Ask the doctor or therapist for his or her opinion as to why this has occurred. And remember the effect is temporary. Relief will follow.

What should I do if the pain increases after treatment?

Should you have the experience of "hurting worse" than before the treatment, be tolerant and patient. Pay attention to how long this effect lasts and report it to your doctor or therapist. Remember: change, however temporary, is a good sign. After a few treatments this therapy reaction will not occur again or with much less intensity.

What should I do to help get the best results?

Do not overuse the area immediately after treatment; allow for the treatment to "absorb" and take effect. In other words, if your damaged knee has just been treated and it feels great, don't go right out jogging. Be sure to follow whatever program of rest or exercise your doctor or therapist recommends.

How many times should I try the treatments if it does not seem to have any effect?

That is between you and your doctor or therapist. Most patients experience obvious improvement by the third or fourth treatment. There are cases on record where the improvement did not start until the eight or tenth treatment. If you have exhausted all other safe methods for pain relief, it is probably wise not to give up before the eighth or tenth treatment. If immediate pain relief is experienced, however temporary, or if there is any noticeable change, of any sort, to any extent, you may be totally pain free long before your tenth treatment with the Electro-Acuscope.

If I have tried many other forms of therapy with little lasting relief, can Electro-Acuscope and Myopulse treatments help me?

Possibly; The Acuscope and Myopulse delivers a different type of treatment than any other form of pain management. It is very often effective where nothing else has been able to help in the past.

My pain seems to be stress-related. Can Electro-Acuscope and Myopulse therapy still help me?

Yes. The therapy is also used for stress management. It can relax the muscles, the nerves, and improve circulation. If you are under excessive stress or your pain is stress-related, your doctor or therapist may apply the relaxation mode in addition to treating directly on the site of pain.

Does this program work for everyone?

No, however most doctors and therapists experienced in its use report that it helps a very high percentage of their patients.

Is the treatment very expensive?

No. Compared to the cost of other pain management programs such as drugs taken over a long period of time and / or surgery, it is quite reasonable.

Will my insurance cover these treatments?

This varies with the type of policy you have. Most private insurance companies cover electrical stimulation. Check with your agent. Ask specifically about the payment policy regarding treatment under the general category of TENS or Electrical Stimulation. Your doctor or therapist may be able to advise you regarding your coverage as well.

Is there anyone who should not be treated?

Under FDA regulations there are two contraindications for use of electrical stimulation. Patients wearing demand-type pacemakers should not be treated. Pregnant patients should not be treated.

CHAPTER 12

SOFT TISSUE INJURIES: TAKING THE MYSTERY OUT OF SPRAINS AND STRAINS

To understand soft tissue injuries, we need to understand a bit of anatomy. The human body is made up of 206 bones which make up the skeleton or hard tissues. Where these bones meet and connect, joints are formed. Connecting these bones and joints are other tissues, primarily muscle and ligaments, which make up the soft tissues of the body. A muscle connects two or more bones to each other and contracts to make the joint move. A ligament also connects two or more bones but functions to limit motion and keep movement within a safe range.

When these tissues are forced beyond their normal range of motion, they can tear. A tear of a ligament is called a sprain and a tear of a muscle is called a strain. Thus, most soft tissue injuries are diagnosed as sprain/strain syndromes. Since ligament tissue has greater density, it usually takes longer to heal, sometimes up to nine months.

Whenever muscles or ligaments are injured, the joints which they support become unstable. Our bodies protect these unstable joints by asking surrounding muscles to contract around them. These muscle contractions or spasms are often referred to as splinting, which is an attempt to prevent the joint and its supportive tissues from further injury by limiting movement of that particular area. The circulation in the injured areas is affected adversely. There is an accumulation of lactic acid and other waste products in the injured tissue, which slows the healing process.

Prolonged pain that lasts several weeks or even months after an injury is usually caused by muscle spasm. The nervous system apparently gets confused and creates its own muscle spasm as a protective response. The spasm that originally started out as part of the normal healing process now becomes its own source of symptoms. The common symptoms are muscle aches, sharp pains in the joints, tension headaches, stiffness and very tender spots in the muscles - sometimes referred to as trigger points.

How do these soft-tissue injuries usually occur?

Automobile accidents are a common cause of soft-tissue injuries. Even minor fender benders can provide enough of a force that can tear the muscles or ligaments. Athletic injuries, any kind of fall, or sudden movement can also cause soft-tissue injuries. Many work related accidents are soft tissue injuries which have involved lifting, pushing, pulling, and slipping, all of which can cause sprains or strains. The other major cause of these injuries, rather than a sudden force, is overuse of the same muscles over a long period of time. For instance, sitting in an incorrect posture day after day at a computer terminal can lead to very similar headaches and muscle aches that a whiplash victim would have.

Within five days after an injury, special cells migrate into the torn fibers and begin to lay down strips of connective tissue called fibrin. These fibrin strands will align themselves along the tear to form a scar and begin to draw the torn edges together. The scar may also attach to other nearby structures, forming an adhesion. This scar tissue patch will be less elastic and weaker than the original tissue, thus predisposing the injured area to future re-injury.

According to the latest research, 90% of all Americans will have muscle aches and stiffness from a previous soft tissue injury. The most common health complaints in America, headaches and back pain, are often related to these improperly healed sprain/strain syndromes.

There is no question that muscle spasms are to blame for most of the common symptoms, but much of the current research is showing that intermingled in this problem with prolonged muscle spasm is the problem of soft tissue adhesion. The early scar tissue fibers don't grow just in line with the tear; they also grow very randomly in other directions and other nearby tissues get; tangled up, so to speak, in the scar. There are many muscles, ligaments, connective tissues and bones that all have to move very smoothly upon each other. When scar tissue forms, adhesions develop which tend to glue and limit tissue elasticity. This leads to all kinds of problems in the way the joints and muscles move.

One of the long term complications of poor joint mobility is that the bones and joints themselves begin to degenerate. Bone spurs, inflammation and arthritis can develop due to this lack of normal joint mobility.

Why can't soft tissue injuries heal on their-own?

When a muscle goes into spasm, it can interfere with it's own blood supply. The spasm crimps off the blood vessels which prevent the waste products of muscle cell metabolism from being carried away and eliminated from the body. This spasm also prevents fresh blood and oxygen from entering the injured area, thus delaying the healing process.

Waste products accumulate and irritate the muscle causing more spasm. The further spasm crimps off other blood vessels which creates an endless cycle of pain and spasm. Many symptoms associated with job related injuries get their start this way. Secretaries, accountants, phone workers and anyone who spends a lot of time in the same position or repeating the same motions will over-use certain muscles. These muscles get irritated, the spasm begins, and once it does, the only thing that can interrupt the cycle is repetitive treatment.

How do you know if you have a soft tissue injury and what is the proper treatment for them?

Even seemingly minor injuries are often more complex than meets the eye. With this new understanding of soft tissue injuries, we now believe that even if someone has a minor injury, which may or may not be causing pain, should have some form of medical treatment to prevent future complications that adhesions might cause.

Orthopedic and neurological tests are often inconclusive since X-rays and MRI's often appear normal. To assess these conditions, the doctor or therapist must pay particular attention to the way a muscle feels and the way a joint moves. Combining this information with the history of the accident and the patient's report of symptoms, a proper diagnosis and assessment can be made.

The goal of treatment is three-fold; first, to relieve the muscle spasm and pain. Second; to both soften the scar tissue and decrease adhesions to ensure that any scar tissue present can move freely over the other nearby tissues. Finally, corrective movement and exercises are taught in order to strengthen and stabilize the areas that are weak and prevent re-injury. To relieve muscle spasms, physical therapy procedures utilizing appropriate electro-therapy and deep-tissue massage techniques help the muscles relax by restoring the normal muscle length, elasticity and resting tone. Stretching and manipulative therapy is also helpful by preventing joints from adhesions and allowing them to function within their full range of motion.

How long does it take to treat these injuries and what health care providers are most qualified to provide the treatment?

It is important to remember that the scar forming across a newly torn tissue takes approximately 8-12 weeks to develop it's maximum strength where it only takes a few days for significant adhesions to take root within the joint capsule. Often times, cases need to be supervised during the initial three month period to make sure that adhesions don't form. In regards to who should treat them, it is usually best to use a team approach. Physical therapy is most successful at relieving the muscle spasm in the early stages. Even within six to eight treatments, much of the spasm and associated symptoms will be gone, even though the scar tissue is still forming. Ideally, treatment should begin as soon as possible and continue through the entire healing period.

Can patients just do exercises at home to keep these scars from forming adhesions?

Home exercises are often a part of a treatment program, but it's usually not enough. There are two reasons for that. First, the muscle spasm has to be treated more aggressively. We have seen, with many years of patient care; that these types of injuries often require a more aggressive approach in order for them to fully resolve and heal. Most people do not have the skills required to safely stretch and relax an injured area. However, these skills can be taught to motivated patients. Other patients may be either de-conditioned or have poor body awareness needed to access areas such as the mid back or abdominal region effectively. Secondly, a specific kind of motion has to be used to treat adhesions. There are three kinds of joint motion. The first is called 'active' and is the motion that can be done by the patient himself with exercise. The second kind of motion is called 'passive' which is performed by a doctor or therapist in order to stretch the joints a little further than the patient can do on their own. In some instances, these types of motion will not affect the adhesion. It is occasionally necessary to provide a third type of motion referred to as a manipulation, which is necessary to free adhesions without injuring the normal tissues. Such a procedure may be necessary to prevent scarring from forming in the joint tissues. That last little bit of motion is the critical difference in treating or preventing adhesions and it is usually performed by someone very skilled in manipulative therapy such as an Osteopath, Chiropractor or Physical Therapist.

Are soft-tissue injuries recognized as a disability for insurance purposes?

At the end of a treatment program, it has to be established whether the patient has reached pre-injury status or whether there's going to be some sort of disability with continuing symptoms. We know from the research that these injuries do not heal with normal ligament or muscle tissue, but instead, they are patched over with scar tissue that may never be as functional and as strong as the original structures. This predisposes the injured area to being more susceptible to future injuries and symptoms. Whether or not that constitutes a case for a liability settlement is difficult to say. The main point from a medical perspective is that these are legitimate injuries, which can cause serious symptoms later and at the very best, increase the likelihood of additional injuries in the future. If the doctors, therapists and the patients themselves take responsibility to see that these injuries are properly treated early on, many complications can be avoided along with unnecessary expense.

What advice do you have for people who believe they might have a soft-tissue injury?

It is important to have your strain or sprain evaluated to determine the extent of the injury and how much treatment may be needed. It is advisable that you consult a health professional who is knowledgeable about soft-tissue problems and the current methods of treatment available such as physical therapy, corrective exercise and manipulative therapy.

Dr. James Cyriax, M.D. author of "The textbook of Orthopedic Medicine," states that many, if not most, of the conditions orthopedic physician's deal with are due to soft tissue scarring from previous injuries. Since there is now a great deal of evidence demonstrating that serious long-term complications are common after apparently minor injuries to muscles and ligaments, it is advisable to seek early intervention. Much of the current pain research has discovered why these problems occur. These research findings recommend an early, aggressive treatment regimen in order to avoid long term complications.

Who uses the Acuscope and Myopulse family of Instruments?

Many health care professionals have trusted and used the Acuscope, Myopulse and Myopulse Facial for over 25 years more than any other instrument. The reason is simple...it works! Athletes like *Michael Jordan, Jack Nicklaus, Joe Montana, Wayne Gretzky, Joan Benoit and Terry Bradshaw* have all had injuries and chronic pain issues. Each of them has been introduced to the Acuscope and Myopulse along with many other celebrities like *Pavarotti, Steven Segal, Lee Majors, Cloris Leachman and Sharon Farret* just to name a few. Veteran golfer Jack Nicklaus, Olympic champions Joan Benoit and Mary Decker, football stars Terry Bradshaw and Joe Montana, hockey great Wayne Gretzky are among the many athletes who have had dramatic results in the resolution of their injuries when they were treated with the Acuscope and Myopulse. Former NFL Football star Terry Bradshaw, used the Acuscope and Myopulse after he severely injured his elbow in one of his games. He says, "After four treatments, I was out of pain and back in the lineup...it's a miracle machine!"

Additionally, the systems have proven to be a superior form of physical therapy and rehabilitation for a wide variety of sport and recreational injuries. Several sports franchises including Toronto Maple Leafs, Philadelphia Flyers, and Chicago White Sox use the Acuscope and Myopulse in their training rooms. Joan Benoit won her Olympic marathon trials only 17 days after arthroscopic knee surgery with a week's worth of treatments with the Electro Acuscope and Myopulse impedance controlled microcurrent systems.

The Equipment: The unique factor which contributes to the outstanding effectiveness of the Acuscope and Myopulse is that the instruments were designed with a proprietary "tissue monitoring" circuitry and "biofeedback" controlled voltage and current waveforms. *In other words these instruments monitor tissue impedance information which is used to carefully control the output current waveform in "real time" as the treatment takes place.*

The Acuscope acts upon subcutaneous tissue and neurological issues to reduce pain and inflammation. It will also improve blood flow in circulatory-impaired tissues. The Myopulse is designed to treat connective tissue associated primarily with muscle, sports injuries, scar tissue and non-surgical facial rejuvenation (Myopulse Facial). The Acuscope, Myopulse Facial and Neuroscope (personal home unit) are effective in restoring the circadian cycles and treating stress, anxiety, addictions and sleep disorders.Treatments are below the "prickling" threshold, are soothing and usually produce significant clinical improvements within the first few applications.

A wide variety of manual hand-held and placement probes have been designed and incorporated into this treatment delivery system including bipolar brass point specific probes, with a variety of precious metal tips for specialty applications, dispersive roller electrodes and large and small placement electrodes for unattended therapy or self-treatment. Specialty probes including: auricular, odonton, lymph drainage, reflexology, soft tissue, facial, cellulite, head band and transcranial ear clips (for head trauma stress, anxiety and sleep) have been designed for health care professionals in every field of chronic pain management, sports injuries and anti-aging esthetics.

Conductive electrolytes, gels and creams are the critical link to the effective utilization of the Acuscope and Myopulse. These complex products are specially formulated to provide accurate two-way communication between the instrument and the tissue, utilizing precious metal and alloy probes as the interface. These electrolytes reduce resistance of the tissue by duplicating the body's electrochemical environment allowing the computers to adjust its current output without interference from the skin. Specialty wound healing and cellulite/stretch mark gels are available as well.

Trusted by all healthcare professionals across North America for over 35 years, the Acuscope and Myopulse have proven themselves to be consistently effective in chronic pain control, trauma rehabilitation, and accelerated healing.

Incorporating the most advanced aerospace technology, these instruments stimulate "tissue repair" rather than "muscle contraction". Utilizing proprietary "carrier wave" technology, the instruments' feedback modulated microprocessors gathers tissue impedance information and in turn provides a gentle current with "waveform control" that accelerates the body's own natural healing abilities. You will experience unparalleled results with the therapeutic effectiveness of the Electro Acuscope, Myopulse and Neuroscope (home care unit). Want to look and feel younger? Check out the Myopulse Facial, a must in today's anti-aging boom! These instruments will consistently surpass all other pain and anti-aging modalities when used to complement your manual therapy and massage skills.

Biomedical Design, the manufacturer of the Electro-Acuscope and Electro-Myopulse, started in 1974 to develop a wide variety of non-invasive, high quality, innovative neuro and muscle stimulating devices. This equipment includes EEG and EMG instruments that monitor bio-conductance of the tissue. Continuous research and development has resulted in amazing breakthroughs in design and effectiveness. New models are offering patients relief from pain and muscle dysfunction beyond what was previously possible because of the advances in microprocessor speeds.

Biomedical Design is a leader in this field and continues to improve the effectiveness of their technology through new probes and conductive electrolyte creams. Muscle reeducation, wound healing and facial tissue regeneration are made possible by advances in software programming and biochemistry.

The Electro-Myopulse 75 was specifically designed to provide today's clinician with an expedient method for treatment of a wide variety of muscle and connective tissue problems. The applications include:

Prevention or retardation of tissue atrophy
Relaxation of muscle spasm
Increasing local blood circulation
Muscle re-education
Maintaining or increasing range of motion
Immediate post-surgical stimulation to prevent venous thrombosis

CHAPTER 13

TESTIMONIALS

"Nine sessions of Physical Therapy with Neil Primack released tension in my upper body to permit continuance of walking and yoga practice, which are essential to my breathing. Now that I am back on my usual routine, my breathing capacity has been significantly improved. Respiratory measurement at the physician's office shows an increase from 17 to 40 points which my doctor rated 'significant.' I am breathing better."

Norma Manson; Kailua-Kona, Hawaii

"My experience with physical therapy by Neil Primack has been healing and uplifting physically and mentally. When I first came to see Neil I was really hurting and depressed for six months from an accident I had in an elevator, where I tripped and fell, ending up with a cervical, shoulder and arm sprain/strain. I would wake up in the morning in so much pain; I didn't want to get out of bed. After only a few months of treatment, I am feeling so much better! I believe the Acuscope and massage therapy that Neil provided has brought a speedy recovery for me." *Carol Rodrigues; Kailua-Kona, Hawaii*

"For about four weeks I suffered with a stabbing pain between my shoulder blades and numbness in my right arm. I couldn't even sleep at night or open a jar with my right hand. Neil was professionally intuitive to the needed therapy to cease my pain and restore strength and feeling in my arm. In just two visits I was comfortable again, and his therapy was relaxing and enjoyable. I looked forward to my physical therapy visit." *Joel Michaelson; Kailua-Kona, Hawaii*

"The treatments I received from Neil Primack were superb. I began my rehabilitation just days after my knee surgery. The benefits showed up immediately and I was able to have my staples removed one week early. Over the past few months I have continued working with Neil using micro-current and exercises. The improvement I've made in my strength and range of motion has been tremendous. The pain has also decreased each week. I'm looking forward to being on the road again soon and being pain free!"

Sean Paget; Kailua-Kona, Hawaii

"For two years I sought treatment for an injury to my neck. Neil is the first of medical doctors, therapists and chiropractors who has been able to zero in on the source of pain and apply his skills to improve my condition. We have been limited by worker's compensation to ten treatments, but even in this short amount of time, I have received the first relief in two years." *Sydney Clough; Kailua-Kona, Hawaii*

"I first saw Neil Primack in the winter of 1991. I had wanted some electro-magnetic therapy for the post-operative pain in my sinuses. Neil took a brief history and then applied the Electro-Acuscope to my sinuses. It took four visits and the pain vanished! Neil also studies a variety of 'vibrational Medicine' systems which I hope to try out in the coming months. As to his personality & character: I have found Neil to be honest, unselfconscious, warm (but not invasive or obtrusive), tactful, pleasant and full of integrity. He is able to establish trust and rapport very quickly. He gives the impression of competence while maintaining a demeanor of modesty. All in all, I highly recommend this therapist."

Margaret Jane Kephart Huizinga; Boulder, Colorado

"I began having severe neck pain about two and a half years ago. I have tried six different chiropractors with six different techniques of adjustment of the neck and spine. At first there would be some relief, but that relief would always be temporary. The pain began returning more and more quickly. I was getting very discouraged by this until I met Neil Primack and began physical therapy with him. He prescribed a therapy that would address not only the muscles of the neck, but of the entire body. His examination found muscle knots throughout my back as well as my neck. These knots had apparently been there for years. They were quite sore to the touch. He said that therapy designed to loosen all these muscles would ultimately clear my neck pain. Since having this therapy there has been a definite improvement in my neck. While I am still not completely free of pain all the time, it is much, much less, and has continued to be less with each visit. I believe that this therapy is the most effective thing I have found in permanently overcoming my neck problem."

Chuck Ceraso; Louisville, Colorado

"I started coming to see Neil in August of 1992. I shattered my cuboid bone in my foot in 1989. This caused me to limp and I started having bad pains in my left knee, hip, back and neck. [I was told] I'd never run, ski, or wear heels. I went to orthopedic surgeons and podiatrists and was told that there was nothing they could do for me and gave me pain pills and said this was a non-surgical injury. I didn't give up. After massage, exercise and Acuscope treatment with Neil, I am no longer taking pain pills and the limping has improved 50%. I can now live my life without being unable to be active and spending so much on doctors. I can't tell you how much Neil has helped me." *Kat Roberts; Boulder, Colorado*

"In 1994, I developed an intense pain in my right hip. I kept thinking that the pain would subside. However, the pain got increasingly worse and began to radiate into my lower back, buttocks and down my right leg. I had a constant headache and got to the point that walking was almost impossible. I was taking 6-8 advil per day for the pain. Finally, in June of 1998, while talking to a friend, she recommended that I make an appointment to see Neil. Neil recommended 10 to 15 sessions of Electro-Acuscope and Myopulse in conjuction with massage. After every treatment with Neil, I could feel I was getting better and better! I stopped taking advil, can now walk without any pain and my headaches completely vanished! I just returned from Europe after 5 weeks, where I walked 5-10 miles a day! Many many thanks, Neil, for all of your help! Because of you, I am able to live a normal life again."   *Susan Bennett; Kona, Hawaii*

"The Acuscope treatments zeroed in on my muscle pain with more pinpoint accuracy and gentleness than the fine elbows of the massage therapist. Now, combining massage with Acuscope is getting the job done! Yeah! The Pilates exercise techniques helped me recover from abdominal surgery more efficiently and gently than several other exercise programs I tried over a year's time. Thank you, Neil, for your help."   *Gail Denton; Boulder, Colorado*

"I was injured in an auto accident and experienced pain and suffering like I never have in all my life. My doctor referred me to Neil Primack. I have since found that my condition has progressively improved through the treatment provided by Neil and his staff. I would summarize my physical therapy with Neil as second to none in the field of health care!"

Curtis Ludwig; Kailua-Kona, Hawaii

ELECTRO-STIMULATION REFERENCES

Extensive literature has been written and scientific studies conducted on the use of micro-current systems to assist in the healing of the body. Specific studies also exist specifically using the Electro-Acuscope and Myopulse systems. An underlying principle of how this equipment operates can be found in the work leading to the 1991 Nobel Price by Dr. Erwin Neher & Dr. Bert Sakmann, demonstrating the effect of ion channels as a means of transporting nutrients into cells. These ion channels are stimulated by one trillionth of an ampere.

Akai, M., et al: Electrical Stimulation of Ligament Healing: An Experimental Study of the Patellar Ligament of Rabbits. Clin. Orthop. ReL Res., 1986, 235:296-301

Assimacopoulos, D: Low Intensity Negative Electric Current in the Treatment of Ulcers oldie Leg Due to Chronic Venous Insufficiency. Am. J.Surg., 1968, 1156823-687

Bassett, CA, Nerriman, I.: The Effects of Electrostatic Fields on Macromolecular Synthesis by Fibroblasts in Vitro. J. Cell. BioL, 1968, 39:9a

Bauer, W.: Electrical Treatment of Severe Head and Neck Cancer Pain. Arch.Otolaryngol - Vol 109, June 1983

Becker, R.O.: Cross Currents; The Perils of Electropollution , The Promise of Electromedicine. Jeremy Tarcher, Inc., 1990

Becker H., Seldon, G: The Body Electric. New York William Morrow & Co., *1985.*

Becker, R., Murry, D.G.: A Method for Producing Cellular DeDifferentialion by Means of Very Small Electric Currents. Trans. N.Y. Academy Sd., 1967 29:606-615

Biedebach, M.C.: A Physiological Model to Explain the Observation of Accelerated Healing and Pain Relief for Computer-Assisted Low Level Electrostunulation. CA: Insutute of Biomolecular Education and Research, 1987

Biedebach, M.C.: Effects of Electro-AcuscopefMyopulse Therapy on Accelerated Tissue Repair. Long Beach, CA. California Stale University

Biedebach, M.C: Many Studies on Microamperage Electrotherapy. P.T. Bulletm. 1988, March 2, p. 5

Biedebach, M.C. : Accelerated Healing of Ischemic Skin Ulcers and the Intracellular Physiological Mechanisms Involved Acupuncture Electrotherapeutics Research, 1989, Volume 14

Biedebach, M.C.: Electro-Acuscope Technology Wave Form Characteristics and Physiological Significance. Long Beach: Dept of Anatomy & Physiology, Preliminary Report, 1989.

Borgens, RB., et al: Electric Fields in Vertabrate Repair. NY: Alan Liss, Inc 2989.

Borslaino, G., et al: Electrical Stimulation of Human Femoral Intertrochanteric Osteotonues. Clin. Orthop. Rd. Res., 1988, 237:256-263.

Bourguignon, Gj., Bourguignon, L.Y.W.: Electrical Stim. of Protein and DNA Synthesis in Human Fibroblast. FASEBJ., 1987, 1:398-402.

Brighton, C.T., et al A Multicenter Study of the Treatment of Non-Union Fractures with Constant Direct Current. J.Bone joint Surg., 1981, A:2-13.

Carley and Wainapel: Electrotherapy for Acceleration of Wound Healing: Low Intensity Direct Current Archives of Physical Medicine and Rehabilitation, Vol. 66, July 1985 Summary: 30 hospital patients with non-healing ulcers were divided into two groups, one treated with conventional wound dressings and one with microcurrent stimulation at 300-700 uA. The latter group was given two hour stimulation periods per day. After six weeks of such treatments, the group treated with microcurrents showed a 150-250% faster healing rate, with stronger scar formation, less pain and lessened infection of the treated area

Cheng, et Al: The Effects of Electric Current on ATP Generation, Protein Synthesis, and Membrane Transport in Rat Skin Clinical Orthopaedics and Related Research, #171, Nov/Dec.1982 Summary: These researchers used in vitro slices of rat skin to determine some of the biochemical explanations for accelerated wound healing demonstrated in the above studies. By applying various levels of current to the samples, and then chemically analyzing them, they determined that skin treated at currents below 1000 uA showed up to 75% higher amino acids and up to 400% more available ATP than controls, and that skin treated at levels above 1000 uA showed depressed levels of of these substances, often less than non-treated controls.

Clark, P.: Forty Niners use Electro-Acuscope for Injury. Oakland Tribune, Jan. 22, 1982.

Curl, D.: Neuro-Electric Feedback Stimulation for Treatment of Temporomandibular Disorders. The American Chiropractor. January, 1988.

Curl, D., Emmerson, G.: The Use of Infa-Red Thermography to Examine the Effects of the Electro-acuscope. Networx-Electric, Sept., 1987.

D'Aloisio, S.: PT Keeps the Famous Up to Par for PGA Tour. P.T. Bulletin. September 17, 1986.

Didomenico, RIL.: Electroacuscope - An Effective Treatment hi Search of a Mechanism. MS/RPT, Physical Therapy Forum, May 4, 1988.

DuPont: Trigger Point Identification and Treatment with Microcurrent, The Journal of Craniomandibular Practice, October 1999, Vol. 17, #4 Summary: This article gives the author's techniques for locating and stimulating trigger points (TP's) using a microcurrent stimulator, specifically for the treatment of temporomandibular disorders. He states that electrical conductivity is highest over trigger points, and galvanic skin response (GSR) testing can be used to locate such points. He utilizes probe electrodes to treat 8pt TP's, and pad electrodes to treat larger ones. Probe treatment is delivered @ 0.3 Hz, 20 - 40 uA, with treatment time of 10 - 30 seconds per site. He suggests administering treatment in 24-48 intervals, and states that results should be seen within 2 - 3 treatments. He acknowledges that these protocols are not necessarily the best ones, but work well for his practice.

F. Rosenberg and E. Postow: Semiconduction in Proteins and Lipids – Its Possible Biological Import," Annals of the New York Academy of Sciences 158 (1969) 161-90

Gersh, M.lt: Microcurrent Electrical Stimulation: Putting It In Perspective. Clinical Management in Physical Therapy, 1989 VoLNo.4, pp.51-54

Gault and Gatens: Use of Low Intensity Direct Current in Management of ischemic Skin Ulcers Physical Therapy, Vol. 56, #3, March 1976. Summary: 100 patients with skin ulcers were treated with microcurrent stimulation; six of them had bacterial ulcers with one side used as controls. Stimulation of 200-800 uA was applied, with negative polarity used until infection cleared, and then polarity reversed. Patients had diagnosis ranging from quadriplegia, CVA, brain tumor, peripheral vascular disease, burns, diabetes, fracture, and amputation. The lesions with patients treated with currents showed approximately twice as fast a healing rate.

Grant, P.: The Use of the Electro-Acuscope/Myopulse System in the Treatment of Chronic Pain: A case study.

Heffernan, M: Comparative Effects of Microcurrent Stimulation on EEG Spectrum and Correlation Dimension, Integrative and Behavioural Science, July-September, 1996, Vol. 31, #3 Summary: 30 subjects were selected for a study comparing the effects of microcurrent on smoothing of EEG measurements of the brain. Subjects were randomly assigned to three groups - microcurrent (100uA) applied to earloble, trapezius area of shoulder, and no stimulation. Electrodes were arranged so subjects could not tell which group they were in. Fast Fourier Transform (FFT) and correlation dimension from chaos analysis were used to measure results. The researcher found that microcurrent applied to the shoulders was markedly more effective in smoothing EEG patterns than earlobe or placebo. "This would represent a possible cost-effective alternative to neurofeedback in treating (anxiety and attention deficit disorders), by raising low regions in the FFT.

Eley, D. D. & Spivey, D. I. (1962) Trans Faraday Soc.58, 411–415

Illingworth, C.M., Barker, A.T.: Measurement of Electrical Currents Emerging During the Regeneration of Amputated Finger Tips in Children. Cm. Phys. PhsioL Meas., 1980, Vol. 1, No. 1, pp. 87-89, Printed in Great Britain

J.A. Spadaro, S.E. Chase, and D.A. Webster: Bacterial inhibition by electrical activation of percutaneous silver implants, Journal of Biomedical Materials Research, Vol. 20, 565-577 (1986) Summary: Percutaneous silver wire implants were placed in rats, and the wounds inoculated with Staphylococcus aureus to test how much infection would spread. Microcurrent stimulation was passed through the wires, with + anodal current placed into implanted silver wire, and the - cathodal electrode placed on the rat's belly as a ground. It was found that significant inhibition of infection occurred, with the most marked results at 20uA current level. "Metallic silver can be effectively and efficiently activated to elicit its anti-microbial activity by the application of microampere electrical current."

Klrsch, D., Lerner, F.: A Double-Blind Comparative Study of Micro-Stimulation and Placebo Effect In Short Term Treatment of the Chromc Back Pain Patient. The ACA journal of Chiropracticf November 1981, VoL 15

Kirsch, D., Madden, K: Low Intensity Transcranial Electrostimulation Improves Human Learning of a Psychomotor Task. American Journal of Electromedicine/ Second Quarter 1987, 41-45

Knoche, V.H.: In Search of a Miracle: Journal of Electro-molecular Medicine. March 1985 VoL 3 No. 1

Lieber,J.: Bradshaw Gets New Hope from the 'Scope. Sports Illustrated, December 19, 1983 Vol. 59, No. 26

Meyers, F.P., Nebrensky, A.: The Electro-Acuscope and Placebo Effect (A Double-Blind Comparative Study in Short Term Treatment of the Chronic Back Pain Patient.) California Health Review, 1983, August/September

Morgareidge, K, Chipman, R.: Microcurrent Therapy. Physical Therapy Today, Spring, 1990.

Noto, K., Grant, P.: Comparative Study of Electro-Acuscope Neural Stimulation and Conventional Physical Therapy Modalities. Physical Therapy Forum, 1985, Vol. IV, No. 11

Nessler and Mass: Direct-Current Electrical Stimulation of Tendon Healing in Vitro Clinical Orthopedics and Related Research, April 1987 Summary: 80 tendons from white rabbits were surgically transected and removed from the animals after being surgically repaired. They were divided into 4 groups of 20, and cultured with 10 of each group being electrically stimulated, and half not. A 1.4 volt direct current connected through a 150 kohm resistor was used for stimulation, at a current of about 7 uA. It was found that currents any higher than this caused discoloration of the tendons. Healing was measured by proline uptake and bridging of the repair site by the epitenon. Results: "a continuous direct current causes, increased tendon cell activity within seven days and the increased activity may persist as long as 42 days." The researchers suggested that externally applied microcurrents may be preferable in future studies.

Oweye, Spielholz and Nelson: Low-intensity Pulsed Galvanic Current and the Healing of Tenotomized Rat Achilles Tendons: Preliminary Report Using Load-to-Breaking Measurements Archives Physical Med Rehab, Vol. 68, July 1987 Summary: 60 rats were divided into three groups of 20. One was unstimulated, one group had their Achilles tendons stimulated with positive (anodal) current, and the third group's tendons were stimulated with negative (cathodal) currents. A current of 75 microamps, at 10 Hz was used. Results: "The group treated with anodal current withstood significantly greater loads (p<0.001) than did either the group which healed normally (i.e. without stimulation) or the group treated with cathodal currents".

Picker, R.L: Low-Volt Pulsed Microamp Stimulation, Part L Clinical Management in Physical Therapy, 1989, VoL 9, No.2, pp. 10-14.

Picker, R.I.: Low-Volt Pulsed Microamp Stimulation, Part II. Clinical Management in Physical Therapy. 1989. VoL 9, No.3, pp. 28-33.

Reichmanis, Marino and Becker: Electrical Correlates of Acupuncture Points IEEE Transactions on Biomedical Engineering, November, 1975 Abstract: Employing a wheatstone bridge, skin conductance was measured over those putative acupuncture points on the large intestine and pericardium meridians lying between the metacarpophalangeal joints and the elbow. Results were compared to those from anatomically similar locations devoid of acupuncture points. "At most acupuncture points on most subjects, there were greater electrical conductance maxims than at control sites."

Richez, Chamay and Bieler, U. of Geneva: Bone Changes Due to Pulses of Direct Electric Microcurrent, Virchows Arch. Abt. A Path Anat. 357, 11-18 (1972) Summary: 26 rabbits had platinum electrodes surgically implanted into the medullary cavities of their humerus bones. Microcurrent stimulation was applied at 50 and 250 uA, allowing pause periods of one second between one second treatment bursts. The scientists found that osteogenesis (bone growth) happened more around the cathode (negative polarity), and that slight tissue necrosis occurred around the anode. The tissues stimulated acted as capacitors, discharging 75% of the current absorbed during the rest periods. They concluded that pulsed current is superior to direct current for bone healing acceleration.

Rossen, J.S.: Microcurrent Stimulation: Why it is Replacing Many Other Forms of Electrical Therapy. The Am. Chiro., 1989, March, pp. 78-82.

Standish, W.D., etal: The Use of Electricity in Ligament and Tendon Repair. Physician Sports Med., 1985, 13:108-116.

Stanish and Gunlaughson: Electrical Energy and Soft-Tissue Injury Healing Sportcare and Fitness, Sept/Oct 1988 Summary: This article is a summary of research into tendon healing acceleration, including human injuries of the anterior cruciate ligament and the Achilles tendons: "While the results are subjective, the individuals in both groups appear to have returned to usual activities more quickly, and have greater mobility, than people treated more conventionally."

Vanable, Joseph: The Role of Endogenous Electrical Fields in Limb Regeneration Limb Development and Regeneration, Part A. pages 587-596 Alan Liss Publishing, N.Y. 1983

Sinitsyn, Razvozva (Russian): Effects of Electrical Microcurrents on Regeneration Processes in Skin Wounds Ortop Travmatol Protez, Feb. 1986 Summary: 68 patients with post burn and post traumatic wounds underwent treatment constant and modulated microcurrent of negative polarity of 1-10 uA/cm2 over a period of 2-20 days. Although both groups showed accelerated regeneration, the modulated electric current group showed more prolonged and marked effect. Better survival of skin grafts was demonstrated compared with untreated patients. Sinitsyn, Razvozova, (Russian): Stimulation of the Regeneration of Skin Wounds by Microcurrents Vopr Juroortol Fizioter Lech Fiz Kult, Nov.-Dec. 1985

Tomoya Ohno (Japanese): Experimental Studies of Influences on Healing Process of Mandibular Defect Stimulated by Microcurrent Shikwa Gakuho, #82 1982 Summary: 50 uA microcurrents were applied to one side of the jaws of a group of dogs with lesions in their jaws. The other side was untreated. The dogs were examined at periods of 3, 7, 14, 21, 28, 42 and 56 days. Results: "It seems likely that direct microcurrent promotes normal bone formation within the defective area and accelerates the osseous healing process. Prolonged application of electrical stimulus promotes a remarkable bone remodeling mechanism."

Wolcott, Wheeler, Hardwicke, and Rowley: Accelerated Healing of Skin Ulcers by Electrotherapy Southern Medical Journal, July 1969. Summary: These researchers applied microcurrent stimulation ranging from 200-800 uA to a wide variety of wounds, using negative polarity over the lesions in the initial phase, and then alternating positive and negative electrodes every three days. The treated group showed 200-350% faster healing rates than control, with stronger tensile strength of scar tissue and antibacterial effects in infected wounds in the treated group.

Thermography and Electrical Stimulation in the Diagnosis and Treatment of Pain By Harold Bess, A.B., D.O., F.A.P.M., Levittown, Pennsylvania. A study of 2,440 liquid crystal thermograms was performed on 206 patients over a period of 26 weeks. Treatment involved the use of the Electro-Acuscope 80 which provides low frequency, galvanic, alternating current to areas demarcated by both the thermograms and the Electro-Acuscope. In myofascial pathology, electrical resistance is increased which delays the healing process and prolongs pain. Regeneration by the Electro-Acuscope is a succession of endothermal and electrochemical biologic reactions. Microscopic amperes of electricity are directed to areas of pain involving tissue pathology to catalyze the regenerative process. The correlation of objective clinical examination findings and liquid crystal thermography was 93%. The correlation between thermography and subjective complaints was 90%. A high correlation of results in identifying areas of injury was noted between thermograms and the Electro-Acuscope. Serial thermograms showed a high correlation with electro-conductivity in response to treatment. Conclusion: Thermography in conjunction with the Electro-Acuscope 80 offers an effective means of diagnosing and treating acute myofascial injuries. Abstract of the 9th International Congress of Physical Medicine and Rehabilitation Jerusalem; May 13-18, 1984

Taubes, G.: An Electrifynig Possiblity, Discover, 1986, April, pp. 23-37.

TRANS-CRANIAL ELECTRO-STIMULATION REFERENCES

Brotman, P.: "Low - Intensity Transcranial Electro - Stimulation Improves The Efficacy of Thermal Biofeedback and Quieting Reflex Training in the Treatment of Classical Migraine Headache " Medical Electronics, Sept 1989

Brown. C. C.: "Electroanesthesia and Electrosleep "American Psychologist, 1975, 30, 402-410

Gibson, T., and O'Hair, D.: "Cranial Application of Low Level Transcranial Electrotherapy vs. Relaxation Instructions in Anxious Patients" American Journal of ElectromedicinelFirst Quarter, 1987

Gomez, E., and Mikhail, A. R. "Treatment of Methadone Withdrawal with Cerebral Electotherapy (Electrosleep)." Brit. J. Psychiatry, 1978, 134, 111-113

Kirsch,D., Madden, K: "Low Intensity Transcranial Electrostimulation Improves Human Learning of a Psychomotor Task." American Journal of Electromedicme, Second Quarter, 1987, 41-45

Kotter, G. S.,Henschel, E 0., Hagan, W J., and Kalbfleisch, J H "Inhibition of Gastric Acid Secretion in Man by the Transcranial Application of Low Intensity PuLsed Current."Gasterocnterology 69 (2) . 3 59-363, 1975

Matteson, J H "The Advantages of Using 'Intelligent' Cerebral Electrical Stimulators in Drug and Alcohol Rehabilitation" Professional Nurses Quarterly, Wmter 1986, p 24

Miller, E W C , and Math.mas, J L "The Use and Effectiveness of Electrosleep in the Treatment of Some Common Psycluatric Problems," American Jour nal of Psychiatry 122 460-462, 1965

Overcash, S. J. and Siebenthall: "The Effects of Cranial Electrotherapy Stimulation and Multi - Sensory Cognitive Therapy on tHEPersonality and Anxiety Levels of Substance Abuse Patients " American Journal of Electromedicine. April 1989. 105-111

Rosenthal, S. H.: 'Alterations in Serum Thyroxine with Cerebral Electrotherapy (Electrosleep) ." Arch Gen Psychiatry, Vol. 28, Jan 1973 Rosenthal, S. H.: "Electrosleep as a Therapeutic Treatment." Comments on Contemporary Psychiatry, July 1971, 1, 25-33

Ryan, J. J. and Souheaver, G. T.: "The Role of Sleep in Electrosleep Therapy for Anxiety." Diseases of the Nervous System,Vol. 38, No. 7, pp 515-517, July 1977

Scaliet, A., Cloninger, C. 8. and Othmer, E.: The Management of Chronic Hysteria: A review and Double-Blind Trial of Electrosleep and Other Relaxation Methods." Dept of Psychiatry, Washington University School of Medicine, St Louis, Missouri, June 1984

Schmitt, R., Capo, T.. Frazier. II. and Boren. D.: "Cranial Electrotherapy Stimulation Treatment of Cognitve Brain Dysfunction in Chemical Dependence."J. Clin. Psychiatry 45: 60-63, 1982

Smith, R. B.: "The Use of Cerebral Electrostimulalion in the Treatment of Alcohol Addiction: A Review." As reported in E. Weingarten, The Effect of Cerebral Electrostimulation on the Frontalis Electromyogram. Biological Psychiatry, 1981, 16, p1

Smith, B. B. and O'Neill, L.: "Electrosleep in the Management of Alcoholism." Biological Psychiatry 1975, 10, 675-680

Smith, B. B. and Day: "The Effects of Cerebral Electrotherapy on Short-Term Memory Impairment in Alcohol Patients." The International Journal of the Addictions, 12(4), 575-582, 1977

Von Richtoffen, C. L and Mellor, C. S.: "Electrosleep Therapy: A Controlled Study of it~s Effectiveness in Anxiety Neurosis." Canadian Journal of Psychiatry, Vol 25, No 3, 213-219, 1980 Weiss, M. F.: "The Treatment of Insomnia Through the Use of Electrosleep: An BEG Study."Journal of Nervous Mental Dis., 157: 108-120,1973

Cranial Electrotherapy Stimulation as a Treatment for Anxiety in Chemically Dependent Persons, Richard Schmitt, PhD, Thomas Capo, BS, Elvin Boyd, MD, Alcoholism: Clinical and Experimental Research, Vol. 10, No. 2, 158-160, 1986

Cranial Electrical Stimulation - CES Reduces Anxiety and Depression, Focus on Alcohol and Drug Issues, Vol. 6, No.1, 1983

Low Intensity Transcranial Electrostimulation Improves Human Learning of a Psychomotor Task, Richard E. Madden, Ph.D., M.S.W.; & Daniel L. Kirsch, Ph.D., American Journal of Electromedicine, 1987

The Use of Cranial Electrotherapy Stimulation in Post-Traumatic Amnesia: A Report of Two Cases, Allen Childs, M.D., M. Lynn Crismon, Pharm.D., Brain Injury, Vol. 2, No. 3, 243-247, 1988

Confirming Evidence of an Effective Treatment for Brain Dysfunction in Alcoholic Patients, Ray B. Smith, Ph.D., M.P.A, Journal of Nervous & Mental Disease, Vol. 170, No. 5, 275-277, 1982

Depression: A Diagnostic, Neurochemical Profile & Therapy with Cranial Electrical Stimulation (CES), C. Norman Shealy, Roger Cady, Robert Wilkie, Richard Cox, Saul Liss, William Clossen, The Journal of Neurological & Orthopaedic Medicine & Surgery, Vo. 10, No. 4, 319-321, 1989

Cranial Electrotherapy Stimulation Treatment of Cognitive Brain Dysfunction in Chemical Dependence, Richard Schmitt, Ph.D., Thomas Capo, Hal Frazier, M.D., Darrell Boren, J Clin Psychiatry, Vol 45: 60-63, 1984

New Treatments Offer Hope for Agitated Brain Syndrome, Allen Childs, M.D., The Psychiatric Times, Medicine & Behavior, September 1988

Electrosleep in the Management of Alcoholism, Ray B. Smith, Lois O'Neill, Biological Psychiatry, Vol. 10, No. 6, 675-679, 1975

Effects of Transcerebral Electrotherapy (Electrosleep) on State Anxiety According to Suggestibility Levels, Joseph J. Ryan, Gary T. Souheaver, Biological Psychiatry, Vol. 11, No. 2, 233-237, 1976

Electrosleep (Electrical Transcranial Stimulation) in the Treatment of Anxiety, Depression and Sleep Disturbance in Chronic Alcoholics, Richard E. McKenzie, Raymond M. Costello, J. Altered States of Consciousness, Vol. 2 (2), 185-195, 1975-76

Changes in Urinary Free Catecholamines and 17-Ketosteroids with Cerebral Electrotherapy (Electrosleep), David F. Briones, M.D., Saul H. Rosenthal, M.D., University of Texas Medical School at San Antonia, Texas, 57-58, 1973

Intracerebral Current Levels in Man During Electrosleep Therapy, A. M. Dymond, R. W. Coger, E.A. Serafetinides, Biological Psychiatry, Vol. 10, No. 1, 101-104, 1975

Treatment of Methadone Withdrawal with Cerebral Electrotherapy (Electrosleep), Evaristo Gomez, Adib R. Mikhail, Brit J. Psychiat., Vol. 134, 111-113, 1978

Electrosleep, A Preliminary Communication, Saul H. Rosenthal, M.D., Norman L. Wulfsohn, M.D., The Journal of Nervous and Mental Disease, Vol. 151, No. 2, 146-151, 1970

Electrosleep: Personal Subjective Experiences, Saul H. Rosenthal, Lynn F. Calvert, Biological Psychiatry, Vol. 4, No. 2, 187-190, 1972

The Effects of Cerebral Electrotherapy on Short-Term Memory Impairment in Alcoholic Patients, Ray B. Smith, Eleanor Day, The International Journal of the Addictions, Vol 12 (4). 575-582, 1977

The Effects of Electrosleep on Insomnia Revisited, Rosalind Dymond Cartwright, Ph.D., Marc F. Weiss, The Journal of Nervous and Mental Disease, Vol. 161, No. 2, 134-137, 1975

The Treatment of Insomnia Through the Use of Electrosleep: An EEG Study, Marc F. Weiss, The Journal of Nervous and Mental Disease, Vol. 157, No. 2, 108-120, 1973

Studies of Electrosleep with Active and Simulated Treatment, Saul H. Rosenthal, M.D., Norman L. Wulfsohn, M.D., Current Therapeutic Research, Vol. 12, No. 3, 126-130, 1970

William A. Tiller, MD. On the Explanation of Electrodermal Diagnostic and Treatment Instruments: Part 1, *The Electrical Behavior of the Human Skin*, Department of Material Science, Stanford University, 1980.

Susan Stockton, *The Terrain Is Everything*, Power of One Publishing, 2000

BIBLIOGRAPHY

"Bioelectronics: A study in cellular regulation, defense, and cancer," Albert Szent-Gyorgyi 1968

"Biologically Closed Electric Circuits" Bjorn Nordenstrom 1983

"Blueprint for Immortality" Harold Saxton Burr, M.D. 1972

"Cross Currents: The Promise of Electromedicine, the Perils of Electro-Pollution" Robert Becker 1990

"Energy Medicine: The Scientific Basis" James Oschman, PhD. 2000

"Membranes Ions and Impulses" Kenneth S. Cole 1972

"Of Animal Electricity" Luigi Galvani 1786

"Rife's World of Electromedicine: The Story, the Corruption and the Promise" Barry Lynes 2009

"The Body Electric: Electromagnetism and the Foundation of Life" Robert Becker & Gary Selden 1985

"The Science Behind Cranial Electrotherapy Stimulation" Daniel L. Kirsch PhD 1999

"The Spark of Life: Electricity in the Humana Body" Frances Ashcroft 2012

"The Prime Cause and Prevention of Cancer" Otto Warburg 1967

"The Secret of Life" Georges Lakhovsky 1929

"The Phenomena of Life; a Radio-Electric Interpretation" George Crile 1936

"Vibrational Medicine" Richard Gerber 2001

ABOUT THE AUTHOR

Neil Primack was born in Monticello, New York in 1960, graduated Fallsburgh High School in 1977 and completed a one year massage program at the Santa Fe College of Natural Medicine in 1982. He graduated from SUNY at Stony Brook with two Bachelor's Degrees in 1986, one in Physical Therapy and the other in Liberal Arts with an emphasis on social science and philosophy. Neil has worked in a wide range of health care settings including: a State Penitentiary, Home Healthcare, Hospitals, Chiropractic offices, Acupuncture Clinics, Medical offices and private practices from 1984 - 2003. He has worked with world class and professional athletes in Boulder, Colorado and Kona Hawaii. Neil has sold and trained numerous health practitioners in the use of the Acuscope and Myopulse including physicians, chiropractors, acupuncturists, physical therapists, nurse practitioners, massage therapists and lay people.

Since 1981, Neil has been a student of Eckankar, an avid reader of books on mysticism, eastern philosophy, and alternative healing. He was trained in The Pilates Method, Positional Release Therapy, certified in Colorpuncture, Kirlian Analysis and various other alternative healing approaches. Since 2004, Neil has been living with his wife and daughter in Jupiter, Florida, where he also assists those looking for help with their Health Insurance and Medicare coverage. Neil enjoys landscaping, film, volleyball and tackling various home improvement projects. He loves sharing insights into Dreaming, Soul Travel, Healing, Past Lives, Reincarnation Mysticism and Mind expansion. There are plans in the works for a Mind-Expansion Studio......Stay tuned.

Neil is the author of two previous books which can be found at: www.amazon.com

"SUDDENLY OUT OF THE BLUE: Insights into life's unique communication from waking dreams and synchronicity" 2016

"BREAKING THROUGH: an autobiographical excursion by way of entheogens, light, sound and dream journey adepts" 2015

For Sales and Training on the Electro-Acuscope and Myopulse please contact Neil at: 561-254-1257 or send an email to: primack@comcast.net

www.ingramcontent.com/pod-product-compliance
Lightning Source LLC
Chambersburg PA
CBHW040807200526
45159CB00022B/46